Praise for *A Guide for Caregiving: What's Next?*

"This *Guide* contains very valuable information particularly for new caregivers. I particularly liked the Self-Care of the Caregiver (Taking Care of Yourself!) chapter."
—*AC, RN*

"I would highly recommend this book for a caregiving class. The very practical tips such as recording things in a notebook, bringing medications to the doctor's appointments and many others—are invaluable and can really make the caregiving tasks easier."
—*CG, Hospital Administrator*

"I believe that two main audiences would use this guide. First and foremost will be the family members coping with the caregiver-caregivee relationship. Additionally, the book would be a good read for healthcare providers, including nurses, physicians, social workers and therapists to understand the scope of the caregiver's work and responsibility."
—*DJ, Physician*

"This *Guide* is a very important source of information for a person becoming a caregiver or those who have been caregivers in the past. There is so much to know! I am a caregiver, and I learned so much. I also think every Doctor's office should have this guide book available to their patients and while waiting in the waiting room."
—*ML, Caregiver*

D1262585

"This is terrific! Not only as a nurse, but also as a family caregiver, I can truly appreciate Tina's insightful guidance provided in this *Guide for Caregiving*. This information would have been a source of much needed insights 15 years ago when I cared for my mother-in-law whose multiple medical conditions were compounded by dementia. It would also have provided much needed direction ten years ago when caring for my mother in her home after suffering a stroke that left her paralyzed on her left side, on tube feedings, and essentially bedridden. And today, as I care for a family member with diabetes and dementia and help a dear friend who requires fourteen prescription medications and a special diet to maintain medical stability. I can rely on this *Guide* for answers to the many issues that I face."

—*Mary St. Pierre, RN, BSN, MGA, former V.P. for Regulatory Affairs, National Association for Home Care & Hospice, Home Care and Hospice Consultant*

"Caregivers of any age or type could benefit from this guide. This includes family members, paid caregivers or aides, and others caring for a loved one or person. I love it—a very much needed resource!"

—*PL, MSN, RN*

"This is such a valuable resource for older adults and their family members!"

—*PZ, RN*

"Tina Marrelli's book is a 'Life Saver.' Worry, doubt, confusion, depression, anger, and feelings of being overwhelmed was what I felt when I realized I was the 'Caregiver.' This book has transformed me into a confident caregiver knowing I could find the answer to most all situations I faced as a caregiver to a loved one and friend. It also made me realize the importance of taking care of myself. I would recommend this book to any professional or any person that find themselves in the caregiver position. It is a valuable tool."

—*Mary Lou Levy, Caregiver*

"None of us are ever ready to be a caregiver. We think we are; especially because we have instructions when leaving the doctor's office or a hospital. Then reality hits and you realize you need help. This Guide gives you that extra knowledge you need. Where to find the resources, support and direction. Every home should have this on their bookshelf!"

—*K. Malloy, Caregiver*

"Being thrust in the position of being cared for or caring for another with medical needs can be daunting and at times overwhelming. *A Guide for Caregiving* is a practical handbook to inspire confidence in the role as an advocate for yourself or your loved one. This knowledgeable resource is a 'must read' to navigate through the maze we call healthcare to provide dignified and compassionate solutions to meet the desired goals of care for yourself or your loved one."

—*Nancy E. Allen, BSN, RNC, CMC Certified Care Manager*

A Guide for Caregiving

What's Next?

Planning for Safety, Quality,
and Compassionate Care
for Your Loved One
and Yourself!

Tina M. Marrelli

Innovative Caregiving Solutions, LLC

NOTICE AND NOTE TO THE READER

To order additional books, buy in bulk, or order for corporate use, contact Innovative Caregiving Solutions, LLC, by emailing tina@e-caregiving.com or (877) 338-3738. To request speaker events schedule, or other media requests, contact the author, Tina Marrelli, at the above e-mail address. If you are a health care organization, this content can also be delivered to your patient population in an e-version. For more information, contact Tina Marrelli at info@ecaregiving.com and visit www.ecaregiving.com.

ISBN: 978-0-692-83608-8

This book is dedicated to Otto Glass. The thoughtful, loving caregiving provided by Bill Glass, my hubby, to his 96-year-old father was exemplary. Dearest Otto, thank you for reminding me that our bodies and health systems are interconnected, and that health care, especially for the chronically ill, the "oldest old" (those over 85), and those moving toward end of life, needs to be thoughtful, supportive, and kind. And that sometimes more care, more experts, and more specialists are not the right thing. The hope is that this book helps others in their caregiving roles as advocate, protector, and expert on their caregivee's care.

Thank you to Cathy Halsey for fun, discussions, and Mr. Jinxs too! Also gratitude to the reviewers, friends, colleagues, neighbors, and others in the throes of caregiving— your input was heard and valued.

Also, to my husband, Bill, and my father, mother, and others who always believed in me.

Contents

Part One
The Caregiver Role:
What the Caregiver Needs to Know   1

Contents

Part Two
Special Patient Populations:
Care Information by Problem 151

About the Author

Tina M. Marrelli, MSN, MA, RN, FAAN

Tina Marrelli is the author of numerous books, including the *Handbook of Home Health Standards: Quality, Documentation and Reimbursement* and her newest book, *Home Care Nursing: Surviving in an Ever-Changing Environment*. She has also contributed regular caregiving columns for over 10 years to newspapers. Tina has personally been a caregiver for a number of years and in that capacity learned that there are skills and duties that can help the caregiver and the person being cared for—the "caregivee." Tina also believes you do not need to be a nurse or other healthcare professional to learn to give care and support to others. This book is the culmination of that belief and experience.

Tina always wanted to become a nurse and help people. To achieve this goal, Tina attended Duke University where she received her undergraduate degree in nursing. She also has master's degrees in health administration and in nursing. Tina has worked in hospitals, nursing homes, and public health settings. She has practiced as a visiting nurse or managed in home care and hospice for many years. Home, for the purposes of this book, is wherever you call "home."

Tina has been married to her "hubby," Bill, for 24 years and hopes for another 24!

Tina is a cat person, but their last one went to kitty heaven (Limpy Buttercup)—so stay tuned for the next kitty! Tina and Bill have done "Sea Turtle Patrol" for over 15 years on the beaches of the west coast of Florida—there is almost nothing as exciting as seeing these vestiges of the dinosaur era come ashore to lay their eggs and then to see and watch their hatchlings, all species of which are either threatened or endangered.

Foreword

As we enter the 21st century, health care presents many challenges—and many opportunities. Change continues to accelerate with new treatments—and new diseases—being discovered at an ever-increasing pace. I have been involved in health care for more years than I want to count. I have been a bench neuroscientist, an academic physician in critical care, a Professor of Medicine at three major U.S. medical schools, a public health professional serving as Director of the Ohio Department of Health, the founder and CEO of a healthcare-related software venture, and, for the past almost 30 years, the founder of a consulting group that has been focused on assisting provider organizations in the post-acute space and governmental agencies to improve the quality of care for vulnerable populations. These groups have included frail elderly patients treated in the skilled nursing facility (SNF) setting, patients treated in home health care setting and in hospice programs, and patients with intellectual and developmental disabilities with significant underlying medical issues.

In 2013, I was developing a plan for a 4-year project working with a large national home health care company and the U.S. DHHS Office of Inspector General (OIG). I was selected to serve as the Compliance Consultant/External Quality Monitor for this project. As the project team was being assembled, I had the very great good fortune to meet Tina Marrelli and then was able to convince her to work with me as a Senior Team Leader for this project.

Tina is clearly one of the most knowledgeable home care experts in the country. She has a long history of ground-breaking contributions to this important and rapidly changing field. Over the ensuing three plus years of working with Tina, I have been continually and increasingly impressed not only by her clinical judgment and knowledge, but also with both the depth of her commitment to meeting the needs of each and every patient she meets and her willingness to think "outside the box" in search of effective solutions to complex and common problems.

Tina Marrelli has been very active working to disseminate best practice information to everyone involved in the care of patients in the home care as well as other settings. This includes, of course, nursing professionals. It also must include patients and families, as Tina recognized in the earliest phase of our understanding of the importance of patient-centered care and the central role patients must play in their decision-making. All disciplines involved, including physicians, social service professionals, skilled therapy professionals, pharmacists and others, must understand the unique aspects of home care and other health care settings. Patient-centered care must include the patient and the family caregivers who provide invaluable caregiving to loved ones, friends, and others.

It is in this context that Marrelli's new book, *A Guide for Caregiving: What's Next? Planning for Safety, Quality, and Compassionate Care for Your Loved One and Yourself!*, represents a very important contribution to understanding how we can all work together most effectively to enhance the quality of care and the quality of life for all involved. Tina always keeps the patient and their family as the central focus for these efforts. Caregivers know their loved one best and are often the "voice" as they advocate for their caregivee's needs.

I highly recommend this new book. It is loaded with practical "nuggets" of information and is very well written. It will be a very useful source of information and guidance for patients/families, nurses, physicians, and all other members of the "team." Caregivers are a very important part of the care team and this book will help them in their quest for quality care, whether in the hospital, at home, hospice, nursing home, assisted living, or other care settings.

David L. Jackson, MD, PhD,
President, Jackson & Associates, Inc.,
Adjunct Professor of Medicine,
Johns Hopkins University School of Medicine

Reviewers

Nancy Allen, BSN, RNC, CMC
Solutions for Care, Inc.
Jacksonville Beach, Florida

Cat Armato, RN, CHPN, CHC,
CHPC, CHPCA
Home Care and Hospice
Compliance Consultant
Blairsville, Georgia

Arlene Chabanuk, MSN, RN,
CDE
Quality Manager
Crozer Keystone Home Health
& Hospice
Springfield, Pennsylvania

Barbara Dale, RN, CWOCN,
CHHN
Quality Home Health
Livingston, Tennessee

Anita Finkelman, MSN, RN
Visiting Lecturer, Nursing
Department
Recanati School for Community
Health Professions
Ben-Gurion University of
the Negev
Beersheba, Israel

Gretchen Riker Gardner, PharmD,
BCACP, CGP
Staff Pharmacist, Rite-Aid
Bremerton, Washington

Calvin E. Glidewell, Jr. FACHE
Former Chief Executive Officer,
Broward Health Medical Center
Fort Lauderdale, Florida

Catherine Halsey, RN, BSN,
CHPN

Dr. David Jackson, MD, PhD
President
Jackson & Associates, Inc.
Adjunct Professor of Medicine
Johns Hopkins University School
of Medicine
Baltimore, Maryland

Kalindi Jackson
Caregiving Consumer
Englewood, Florida

Mary Lou Levy
Caregiving Consumer
Venice, Florida

Paula Long, MSN, RN
Clinical Director
Home Health Care
Clinton, Indiana

Donna Lucci, OTR/L
Registered Occupational Therapist
Encompass Home Health
North Reading, Massachusetts

Jessica L. McDevitt, PT
Wakefield, Massachusetts

Mary McGoldrick, MS, RN, CRNI
Home Care and Hospice Consultant
Home Health Systems
St. Simons Island, Georgia

Kathleen "Katie" Mayme Malloy
HealthCare Consumer and Caregiver
Venice, Florida

Sandra Whittier, MSN, RN
Home Health Geriatric Nurse
Swampscott, Massachusetts

Patricia Zabell, RN, BS, MBA, CHCE, HCS-D, COS-C
Interim Leader
B. E. Smith
Sarasota, Florida

Preface: People Do Not Live in the Hospital!

This book began when I saw older friends being discharged from health care systems or hospitals. I noted that they were being sent home with a lot of information—some of it very useful and some, not so much. And what good is it, really, if someone has multiple health problems and they are given four booklets—one for each health problem? This recently happened to a friend of mine who was discharged from the hospital. This means if you have diabetes, heart failure, and chronic obstructive pulmonary disease (COPD), you are sent out with three (or more, depending) 20-plus page booklets. As we age, the complexity of chronic health care conditions can also increase, which could make this a very problematic answer to informational, care-management needs.

Because I am a registered nurse and have been writing newspaper columns for many years about caregiving, it became apparent that this information was needed. There has got to be a better and more understandable way to help people connect the dots related to health and health care! The information I saw sometimes sliced and diced their health care problem(s) and made their care try to fit into an unrealistic "one size fits all" model. I am old-fashioned and believe in the wisdom of the body. Nurses are particularly adept at helping people and their unique responses to both health and illness. As health care has become more specialized and

complex—we have lost some very dear and important concepts. The most important concept we have lost is the person
as an individual. We—you and I and others—all together
need to reframe and help to reshape healthcare. We need
to become the voice—not a TV show—but a thoughtful,
activated, and committed group of health care professionals,
consumers, and caregivers who contribute positively, each
in our own way, to our communities, to help make health
care the way we want it to be. This book hopes to contribute
to this community-based effort that will move us toward
a prevention-focused model of care with the patients and
caregivers at the center. One measurement for knowing this
transformation has been successful is that the primary care
provider or doctor would also ask the caregiver accompanying
the patient how they are doing, and perhaps even checks their
blood pressure.

Some of this is so fundamental—both from being a nurse
and from personal experience, living with a 96-year-old
person in my own home for some years! This means that
sometimes it does not matter what the 96-year-old caregivee/
loved one "has wrong" with him; it is all about what matters
to him! How frailty limits movement and speed, how the loss
of long-term friends is painful, and such functional things as
forgetting to take pills, remembering to use a cane, see their
glasses to find them (to put them back on), and much, much,
more. This book is an attempt to answer many of the questions and concerns that family and other caregivers, such as
aides, have asked over the years.

This book is also a call to improve end-of-life care. As of
2016, Medicare covers "advance care planning," conversations about end of life care toward end of life plans with

practitioners (PBS, 2016). We know we will be there and need this—but what does the best and most compassionate care "look like?" These important questions need to be addressed across the life span—it is never a one and done. This needs to be a thoughtful discussion with a healthcare professional who knows you and, as importantly, your wishes to help you and your family to develop a plan that honors and respects these choices. Sadly, much care is provided at end of life that perhaps would not be chosen had more discussion(s) and education occurred before a "crisis" happened. We all need to work on communication and coordination skills in this area. The article from *The Atlantic* by Dr. Angelo Volandes called "How Not To Die" skillfully presents about the need to revolutionize care at end of life (http://www.theatlantic.com/magazine/archive/2013/05/how-not-to-die/309277/). In this article, the author talks eloquently about the conversation and those areas of care that need more transparency, education, compassion, and understanding to improve care at this special time that we all will experience.

Let's step back—picture the best vision of the future for healthcare. In that new improved healthcare world, there are only terms used that a "lay" person or non-healthcare professional can understand! If there is one goal for health care professionals in this book, this is it—that we explain terms in understandable words. This is not asking too much. It is also important that health care professionals across all settings help to support and honor that choice when people want to be cared for at home.

From practicing as a long-time home care nurse (after years of inpatient settings), it is easy to understand why people want to be cared for at home. This is where healthcare gets most personalized, wishes are more easily honored, and, for numerous reasons, it is where many people prefer to be and live out their days—including care at the end of life if this is chosen and possible. Home care has no limits on the visiting hours, the age of visitors, the music played or the volume of that music, there may be pets that live there and are often a source of great comfort, the food is great, the clothes are much better (though I heard that Diane Von Furstenberg is creating hospital gowns!), and numerous other reasons. There truly is "no place like home."

The movement toward home care and the provision of health care at home also brings health care back to its roots—where healthcare was delivered in communities and much care was provided with skill and compassion in the home, and most often by loved ones, friends, and family with the support of the community nurse. Home care, palliative care, and hospice need to be the fundamental framework for health care. It is well-known in reported research that this is where people wish to be cared for.

This book hopes to bring back the fundamental understanding that health care and people are and should be interrelated and interconnected. These concepts support and inform proactive care. As I sometimes say lovingly in my caregiving columns in newspapers—Think of the old song: "the hip bone's connected to the thigh bone." This fundamentally means that our body systems are interrelated and interconnected. This is why there are 12 Special Patient Population Sections including "Alzheimer's Disease and Dementia Care," "Arthritis Care," "Bedbound Care (Care of the Immobilized or Bedridden Patient)," "Cancer Care," "Cardiac Care," "Diabetes Care," "End-of-Life, Palliative, and Hospice

Care," and others. In this way, there is one book to help you navigate caring for your loved one. Caregiver readers can refer to various areas for more information and this information was specifically designed to provide an easy reference to individualize care while supporting the interconnectedness of health and healthcare.

It should go without saying that patient and caregivers should adhere to and/or be compliant with health care regimens recommended by their health care providers. In fact, not adhering to recommendations has caused patients to have poorer health and outcomes. Health care providers might also want to be aware that some people (really!) do not understand why they should not smoke, be obese, eat a lot of sugar, or drink alcohol to excess. This nonadherence also contributes to increased health care costs. In this book, "provider" can refer to a number of professionals. This may include the physician, nurse practitioner, physician assistant, a registered nurse, a scribe (a person who documents the care provided), medical technician, the hospitalist, or any number of people involved in the care. Whatever your health care provider's title might be, it is imperative that patients/consumers and caregivers know who is caring for them. For example, lots of people wear white in hospitals—including lab coats—but is the person a nurse, or a registered nurse (RN), or perhaps a lab technician? It is very important that a patient knows who is caring for them!

The other goals of this book are that patients and consumer caregivers become empowered to care for loved ones and others in all care settings. In this model, they know everything there is to know about their caregivee/loved one and are active participants in care, care planning, and discharge.

Often, it is the patient/caregiver team who are the "experts" on the care needs of the patient.

I envision a healthcare world where the caregiver comes into the hospital with the patient to participate in, contribute to, and continue to care for the patient even after they leave the hospital. I hope caregivers will be able to provide important input and be seen as core parts of the care team. I know this well from practicing in home care, that hospitals and other care settings need to recognize and embrace what is a great and tremendous source of information and care—the caregiver, often a family member! This is all in an effort to better coordinate, communicate, and standardize care across care settings; for example, when the patient must go into the hospital from the home setting and then returns back to the home. The one constant is that very important caregiver or patient representative. Working with committed caregivers is one answer to improving safety and quality in health care. I challenge hospitals and other inpatient providers to embrace this untapped and special workforce!

Reference

PBS. (2016). 5 things you should know about Medicare's new end-of-life discussions. Retrieved from http://www.pbs.org/newshour/making-sense/5-things-you-should-know-about-medicares-new-end-of-life-discussions/

How to Use This Book

The goal of this book is to assist caregivers as they care for their caregivee/loved one. Keep in mind that there may be more than one section that is applicable to your caregivee/loved one's health needs. For example, when caring for someone with both cancer and who is at the end of life, you may wish to refer to "End-of-Life, Palliative, and Hospice Care" as well as "Cancer Care." In some sections of the book there are references to other sections that also may be helpful.

Part One—The Caregiver Role: What the Caregiver Needs to Know—Part One is comprised of ten chapters. These chapters are specially designed to provide an overview of a specific area of caregiving. These chapters provide fundamental knowledge about caregiving and being a caregiver. Readers are encouraged to read the parts of the book that are of immediate interest to them—however, please understand that the book was specifically designed to build on the knowledge base of the prior chapters. To this end, it is recommended that readers progress from Chapter One through Chapter Ten. In addition, should your hospital or care system use this book as a text or supplement to their caregiver classes, they may direct you to read certain sections that are of particular importance for the safe and effective care of your loved one/caregivee.

Part Two—Special Patient Populations: Care Information by Problem—Part Two is comprised of 12 care sections, listed and organized according to the health care problem. These are listed and organized alphabetically, for ease of finding and using the information as needed. The care information listed in Part Two is all in a standardized format. The sections are:

1. **Introduction**—This first section provides information, data, and/or statistics about that specific care problem. These numbers help caregivers know they are not alone! Each chapter starts with a definition, and statistics are provided where applicable. For example, in "Alzheimer's Disease and Dementia Care," which is the first care problem alphabetically, it states that "research reported by the National Institute on Aging suggests that as many as 5 million Americans have Alzheimer's disease, although estimates about that number vary." Please know that the statistics chosen are the most up-to-date and from well-known and credible government or other expert sources at the time of publication.

2. **General Information**—This section provides specific information about the health problem being addressed. Using "Alzheimer's Disease and Dementia Care" as an example, one of the best known difficulties in the care for a caregivee/loved one with Alzheimer's Disease (AD) is that it is very stressful because of the 24-hour nature of the care needed. This section might also refer the reader to other relevant sections in the book. Again, using AD as an example, the reader is referred to Chapter Eight: Self-Care of the Caregiver (Taking Care of Yourself!) because of the

time and commitments required when caring for a person with AD.

3. **General Goals for Care**—This section identifies in clear, "bottom-line" terms the goals for care. Using the AD example again, there are two goals—one for the caregivee/ loved one and another for the caregiver. In this way, the direction of the care is prioritized from a safety and quality perspective. The goals are fundamental and clearly written. This section continues with the usual goals and activities for specific health concerns and problems to support health and safety.

4. **Personal Care Considerations**—Personal care in this book refers to bathing and other activities of daily living that are generally accomplished every day to support hygiene and health. This section may also include tooth brushing, dressing, laundry, meal preparation and serving, and many other activities and tasks. Anything specifically related to personal care and the problem being addressed would be listed in this section. Again, using the AD example, some people with AD do not like water or to shower or take a bath. Such information and tips to make this process safe and enjoyable for all involved would be listed in this section.

5. **Safety Considerations**—This section clearly lists aspects of certain problems and their safety-related challenges. Using the AD example, one safety consideration that should be watched for would include wandering behaviors.

6. **When to Call the Doctor, Nurse, or Care Team**—This section lists when the care team should be called. There is no way to list ALL the possible problems that can

occur—that is why it is so important that care be individualized and that the caregivee/loved one is closely monitored during care. This is a list based on the particular problem. When in doubt, call your health care team member!

7. **Comfort Considerations**—This section is comprised of the things the caregiver can do to provide comfort to the caregivee/loved one. This section takes a proactive, "holistic" approach to care. Holistic means that the whole person is seen and cared for—this includes the mind, body, spirit, and other dimensions of caring and health. For purposes of this book, physical, mental, and spiritual aspects of a person are addressed. This might include a back rub, time spent with a beloved pet, or a drive to see a sunset or sunrise. These are suggestions to consider, directed toward and related to comfort, which can be a part of anyone's daily care and life.

8. **Special Considerations**—These are special considerations or information that should be considered for your caregivee/loved one's unique care problem(s). These are ideas to think about from a long-term perspective and to help the caregiver identify when there might be a need to make a change or reevaluate the care, a related care process, or care setting.

9. **Special Instructions Given to You by the Doctor, Nurse, or Care Team**—These are a series of blank lines so that you or your care provider, such as a doctor or nurse, can write down anything special for you about your caregivee/loved one's care. This section may also be completed by the clinic or discharge planner who gave you this book or the nurse who may be providing specific teaching. It is

recommended that if this book is given to you when being discharged from a hospital, that the date and time of your caregivee/loved one's next doctor or other health care appointment be written here.

10. **Resources for You**—This section lists web sites and other (usually) free, government or other resources that may assist you in your caregivee/loved one's care. In the example of AD, this might include the National Institute on Aging's website on AD, the Centers for Disease Control and Prevention site dealing with AD care, and other science-based sources of more information to help the caregiver become more knowledgeable about a health problem and to be able to anticipate changes by knowing the trajectory and usual course of AD, for example.

Part One

The Caregiver Role
What the Caregiver Needs to Know

Chapter One

The Caregiver Role:
Overview of a Very Important Role

You may have bought this book or been given this book because you are or will be a caregiver. Or you might be the primary caregiver and you may need to find and hire aides or other caregivers when you need to be away or need a break. Whatever the reason—I understand and you are not alone!

In fact, according to a 2014 report commissioned by the National Institutes of Health (NIH), America's older adult population is "now over 40 million and expected to more than double by mid-century, growing to 83.7 million people and one-fifth of the U.S. population by 2050" (National Institute on Aging [NIA], 2014).

If you take a walk down your street, shop at the grocery store, go on a cruise, wait at a boarding gate at the airport, or generally are out in public—you can see that we are all aging. This is also seen in the increasing numbers of canes, walkers, wheelchairs, and scooters we see used in society. Taken together, this information shows that caregiving will continue to increase. In addition, as society ages, so too may the complexities of care and caregiving.

The intent of this book is to help support you by providing you with information and other resources to help you be/become an empowered, engaged caregiver as well as an advocate for your family member or for those for whom you provide care. And, as important, to be able to harness those skills and bring them with you when you accompany your loved one or "caregivee" to the doctor, nurse practitioner, emergency department, or wherever else you may go for health care. For purposes of clarity, the person receiving the care will be called the "caregivee." This same person may be a spouse, your loved one, a sister, best friend, lover, or others needing care. Sometimes a non-family member or a paid caregiver may be the caregiver. This may be a lay person, such as a friend, a credentialed home health aide, or other person, such as a nurse. This all depends on the patient or caregivee needs, the environment of care, and other circumstances. Professional or specially-trained caregivers may be home health aides, home care aides, hospice aides, certified nursing assistants, personal care aides, or others.

What is a Caregiver and Who are Caregivers? A Fundamental Definition

People from all walks of life can become and are caregivers. Because most people report that they wish to remain at home, much caregiving is provided in the home. Hospital stays or days of care are getting shorter and more care has moved outside the hospital. All these factors make the home an important setting for care and caregiving.

There are many definitions for caregivers and caregiving. For purposes of clarity, here is a fundamental one–especially since data show that it is oftentimes family who provide the care: "family caregivers may be spouses, partners, children, relatives, or friends who help the patient with activities of daily living and health care needs at home" (National Cancer Institute, 2013). I first became a caregiver when my (at that time!) 96-year-old father-in-law moved in with my husband and me. And we became caregivers!

As you may have also learned or seen, many older adults, particularly the oldest-old, who are defined as people age 85 and older (NIA, 2011), have many personal care and safety needs because of their advanced age. As a home care nurse for many years, I have helped many families grow in their comfort and skills to help their loved ones at home. Many major contributions to society have been made by people considered the oldest old. Keep in mind that there is a difference between biological and chronological age.In addition, I have written a "Caregiver Column" for some years for newspapers. In this column, family members or friends who are caregivers, have written to me about their specific concerns and questions. Through all these questions, I have learned the depth and broad range of families, friends, and their caregivers.

Getting Old is Not an Easy Process—Some Numbers

As a registered nurse, I have heard this statement from many patients across the years. Some have survived life-threatening illness such as cancer or trauma and/or have increased frailty or other health problems from treatments. Whatever the loved one's/caregivee's unique health problems and history, caregivers, especially family, are being asked to provide more and more care. This trend is not expected to change. In fact, Medicare, the largest payer of health care services for older adults, is working toward decreasing unneeded, and very costly, rehospitalizations when possible. Patients in the Medicare program are not getting younger. In fact, life expectancy at birth for the United States U.S. population reached a record high of 78.8 years in 2012 (Centers for Disease Control and Prevention [CDC], 2014). For males it was 76.4 and for females it was 81.2 years (CDC, 2014). In addition, there were 49 million Medicare beneficiaries in 2012 (The Henry J. Kaiser Family Foundation, n.d.). Medicare is a complex medical health insurance program for those 65 and older, those who are disabled, those who have End Stage Renal Disease (ESRD), and those who meet a few other criteria. For more information on Medicare, visit www.Medicare.gov or visit your local Social Security office. This increased age leads to increased personal care needs (such as bathing) and activities of daily living (ADLs) (such as eating, shopping) needs. It is caregivers who must assume or arrange for these important and numerous needs in order to support health and safely maintain the caregivee in the home.

Aging and Health Care: A Snapshot

In 2013, the 65 and older age group represented 14% of the U.S. population (United States Census Bureau, 2014). It is estimated that by 2030 nearly one in five persons will be aged 65 and older (NIH, 2006). Safety and falls are always a concern when addressing the health needs of older adults, as well as children. Emergency department visits are one snapshot of this growing problem. According to NCHS Data Brief No. 130, twenty-nine percent of Emergency Department (ED) visits by persons aged 65 and over were related to injury and the percentage was higher among those aged 85 and over than other age groups of older adults (United States Department of Health and Human Services, 2013). It was also found that the percentage of ED visits caused by falls increased with age. This is important because the ED is a venue that may lead to hospitalization for many Medicare patients. This book and its information will help you navigate to try and avoid, when possible, stressful and sometimes unnecessary ED visits. Most EDs are not a welcoming or comfortable place for older adults. We hope the information in this book helps and empowers you to ask your doctor when you have questions about the ED and, perhaps, about making home visits, or other, better ways to care for older adults where they often live—at home.

Increasing Complexity of Care

As health care has become more specialized, it has also become more fragmented and, sometimes, more confusing. And, as mentioned previously, the world is aging, and there are also many old and sometimes very old caregivers. It is not unusual to see an 80- or 90-year-old caregiving for their spouse of the same age and this is a continuing trend. There are a number of reasons for this, but this has many important implications for caregivers. What this means practically is that more and more of our friends and ourselves will be having complex and chronic diseases as we age. An example of this chronic and complex care is that the person does not have only one diagnosis or health problem, such as diabetes. They may also have cancer, high blood pressure (also called hypertension), heart problems or wound/skin problems on their lower legs, and more. Along with these multiple conditions may come multiple medications. Medications in older adults, especially frail individuals, can pose their own risks and concerns. It is for this very reason that this handbook is easy to use. The reader(s)/caregiver(s) can easily switch to those sections of the book that address your unique situation, as needed. Your healthcare team are resources for your questions and answers that pertain to your particular situation. In fact, you are encouraged to have an ongoing relationship with a health care professional such as a doctor or nurse practitioner or others as needed. This information is in no way a substitute for your doctor's or other health care professional's instructions. They know you and your caregivee/loved one's unique situation and care needs. In addition, it is important to note that the caregivee/loved one and their caregiver are the expert on themselves and their day-to-day concerns.

Caregivers themselves must provide their own "self-care" to be effective caregivers and care for themselves (more about this in Chapter Eight: Self-Care of the Caregiver [Taking Care of Yourself!]).

Now that the definition of the caregiver is known, the next chapter addresses the unique skills needed to be a good and effective caregiver.

Summary

This chapter summarizes the aging demographic of the United States and the corresponding need for family and other caregivers. Many of us will become or are already caregivers in some capacity. This first chapter seeks to clarify terms and provide examples to overall help you help the care team of doctors, nurses, and others caring for your caregivee/loved one. You are not alone!

Resources for You

- The U.S. Department of Veterans Affairs offers a Caregiver Support page: http://www.caregiver.va.gov/toolbox/index.asp
- USA.gov offers caregiver resources including locating tools for finding care, assisted living, home care agencies, hospices, and more at their Caregivers' Resources page: http://www.usa.gov/Citizen/Topics/Health/caregivers.shtml
- The National Institute on Aging offers a booklet called Long-Distance Caregiving: Getting Started that discusses how you can play a role even if you do not live close to the person needing care: http://www.nia.nih.gov/health/publication/long-distance-caregiving-getting-started

References

Centers for Disease Control and Prevention (CDC). (2014). Mortality in the United States, 2012. Retrieved from http://www.cdc.gov/nchs/data/databriefs/db168.pdf

National Cancer Institute. (2013). Family Caregivers in Cancer. Retrieved from http://www.cancer.gov/cancertopics/pdq/supportivecare/caregivers/patient/page1

National Institutes of Health (NIH). (2006). Dramatic changes in U.S. aging highlighted in new census, NIH report. Retrieved from http://www.nia.nih.gov/espanol/newsroom/2006/03/dramatic-changes-us-aging-highlighted-new-census-nih-report

National Institute on Aging (NIA). (2014). NIH-commissioned Census Bureau report highlights effect of aging boomers. Retrieved from http://www.nia.nih.gov/newsroom/2014/06/nih-commissioned-census-bureau-report-highlights-effect-aging-boomers

National Institute on Aging (NIA). (2011). Why Population Aging Matters: A Global Perspective. Retrieved from http://www.nia.nih.gov/health/publication/why-population-aging-matters-global-perspective/trend-3-rising-numbers-oldest-old

The Henry J. Kaiser Family Foundation. (n.d.). Total Number of Medicare Beneficiaries. Retrieved from http://kff.org/medicare/state-indicator/total-medicare-beneficiaries/

United States Department of Health and Human Services. (2013). Emergency Department Visits by Persons Aged 65 and Over: United States, 2009–2010. NCHS Data Brief No. 130. Retrieved from http://www.cdc.gov/nchs/data/databriefs/db130.pdf

United States Census Bureau. (2014). State & County QuickFacts. Retrieved from http://quickfacts.census.gov/qfd/states/00000.html

Chapter Two

Skills Needed to Be a Good Caregiver

You may already know some caregivers. Perhaps their older adult parents are living with them. Or they may have a child with special needs who needs care at home. Whatever the unique situation, the caregiver has many responsibilities, tasks, and roles related to taking care of the adult or child needing care.

Let's look at three examples.

1. A 67-year-old man is discharged from the hospital with a long history of diabetes (a disorder characterized by high blood sugars and other health problems) and obesity (he weighed 290 pounds when last weighed at the hospital), and is coming back to his home after a long hospitalization that started with chest pain and, as he reported, "heart problems." He no longer drives and is also depressed. His adult daughters received a phone call from the local hospital discharge planner explaining that their father is being sent back home, with discharge planned for the next day, but needs some specialized care such as medication management. He is also being sent home with a new special diet, a recommended gradual exercise program, and more lifestyle changes. Their father will also need to come back to the hospital's outpatient department for ongoing education about diabetes management and care. The daughters

are also encouraged to attend. The daughters can see that their father can no longer function safely on his own.

2. A child was born with health problems (called congenital) and cannot walk or eat or feed himself nor participate in many of the other mobile play activities that most other 4-year-olds can perform. There are specialized nurses, aides, teachers, and therapists who help care for him. Still, the parents are in the home and there are two other children, aged 6 and 2, as well. These parents, though they may also have others coming in to help care for their child, are caregivers. Their daily activities, and oftentimes their lives, revolve around the needs of this child's very complex care. They can become isolated and exhausted in this routine that may continue for years.

3. A 97-year-old woman moves in with her adult daughter and her husband. Though the mother is very thin and "frail," she can still walk with some assistance and the use of a cane. The mother needs help to shower, needs her meals prepared and "set up," and needs help and assistance with other components of personal care and activities of daily living. She is also very forgetful and so cannot cook on the stove. The daughter and her husband's schedules have been adapted to make this situation work. They get up at the same time every morning and prepare her meal, serve the meal, make sure that (the correct) medications are "poured" and taken, that Mother brushed her teeth, is dressed cleanly and appropriately for the weather, and the many other things that we all must do to maintain personal hygiene and to "get ready" for the day. They notice that Mother's forgetfulness is increasing and that she left the bathroom sink faucet on with water running

twice last week—one time with the water running out of the sink bowl and onto the floor and starting to go down the stairs. Luckily, they were home that day—they usually both work, though. They wonder how long they can manage her care needs as her condition deteriorates.

The sad fact is that it is likely that some of these chronic situations do not get better—unfortunately, they sometimes get more problematic and unsafe and sometimes become unmanageable at home.

Though very different circumstances, what these situations have in common is the commitment to caregiving and trying to make things "work" for all involved. I have had people say to me "I could not/never bring my mom or dad or _____ (complete the blank with family, friend, or loved one that you could not imagine living with) to live with us—they are too difficult, demanding, or otherwise not a good candidate to bring home!" Sometimes, the house has too many steps or other situations that may not be safe for care at home. With this in mind, remember not all people can be brought home or stay home, even with support and care and the best of intentions. The following are some questions to ask yourself as you think about being/becoming a caregiver.

The Caregiver's Checklist for Consideration— Questions That May Help in Determining What is Best for Your Caregivee/Loved One

Note: There are no right or wrong answers. This is a hard topic to discuss because not everyone can be cared for at home. This can be for many reasons. In addition, there may be guilt, either self-guilt or guilt placed on you by outside persons, when the decision is made by all involved that home caregiving is not or is no longer an option. Some people have this guilt even when they have to place someone in an institution or rehabilitation center for the safety of the caregivee/loved one. These statements and areas of consideration are just a few ways to help you judge your interest, commitment, abilities, and capabilities for success in this role.

Space/home considerations:

- Does the space and physical characteristics of your home support safety in caregiving?
- Do you have a separate space for your caregivee/loved one to stay/sleep?
- Is your home appropriate for caregiving? From a safety perspective, this might include level floors and/or no stairs (or chair or elevator access to those levels).
- Are there hand rails on stairs for assistance to get in and out of the home?
- Are there bathrooms with safety features?
- Is there heat and air conditioning in the home? This is especially important if the person needing the care has respiratory conditions such as asthma and/or COPD.
- Is there running water and hot/warm water for bathing, hand washing, and other infection control and comfort activities?
- Is there room for a hospital bed (such as downstairs) if the person can no longer sleep upstairs?
- Oxygen is sometimes used at home. Are there smokers in the house? NO SMOKING can occur when oxygen is in

the home and be aware of other open flames, such as gas stoves.

- If/as the caregivee/loved one progresses in the home, is the home accessible to a wheelchair? Are the doorways wide enough for a wheelchair to pass through safely?

Interpersonal considerations:

- Who else lives in the home? Are others understanding of your caregivee's/loved one's needs? Are they empathetic? A positive attitude and space is very important in the home environment to help healing, comfort, and overall health of sick persons.
- Privacy considerations include the actual space, the ability to have a private conversation, etc. One caregiver reported to me that what she missed most was the ability to go get a cup of coffee in her nightclothes as her father-in-law was always awake and in his "TV chair" before she woke up— so the consideration of a lack of quiet time/space/alone time is an important one.

Interpersonal and "can-do" considerations and attributes needed:

- Patience
- Kindness
- A caring manner
- Effective listening skills
- A schedule that can be flexible/adapted to the needs of the caregivee/loved one
- A positive attitude and a good sense of humor
- An understanding of the importance and practice of effective hand washing and other infection control-related activities

- An understanding of comfort measures (such as massage, positioning for comfort, and/or playing cards or music with caregivee/loved one)
- Ability to care sensitively and compassionately for caregivee/loved one, especially at the end of life
- Empathy and understanding
- Organizational skills (may include scheduling doctor visits, hair appointments, senior center activities, obtaining private care, organizing visiting nurse association (VNA) services, or others as unique as your caregivee/loved one)
- Knowledgeable about and resourceful in obtaining durable medical equipment or other supplies as needed.

Sample Caregiving Activities

- Strong safety awareness ("see" items such as throw rugs, clutter in walkways, open dishwasher door that a frail older adult may not see and trip on/over, pets, etc.)
- Observation and reporting skills
- Hands-on activities, such as assisting with personal care like bathing, hair, skin, nail care, and shaving
- Mouth and oral care
- Catheter/other tube care
- Advocacy skills or the ability to speak about and speak up for your caregivee/loved one's needs
- Can follow healthcare-related instructions/direction
- Toileting care and writing/keeping track of caregivee/loved one's activities, such as urination (peeing) and bowel movements (BMs)
- Medications—ensuring that they are the correct medication, the dose is correct, the ability to help the patient

adhere to the regimen, and ensuring that there is access to get the medications, such as transportation or getting them delivered

- Care of the bedbound person (perhaps possible or eventually if not now)
- Awareness of changing mood or depression
- The physical ability to assist/turn/lift/support/transfer the caregivee/loved one
- Awareness of the caregivee/loved one's psycho-spiritual considerations.

Assistance with activities of daily living:

- Shopping, meal planning
- Meal preparation, cooking, and serving
- Ambulation assistance
- Assistance with walker, cane, wheelchair, other assistive devices
- Laundry activities and assisting with dressing
- Ongoing grooming, bathing, and hygiene-related activities

Others:

- Attendance to doctor visits
- Home exercise program provided by health care team
- Application/assistance with elastic or support stockings/ hose
- The use of proper safe body mechanics
- Housekeeping activities
- Cards, church, or continued connections with support systems, friends, clergy, and/or other activities
- And others, too numerous and individualized for the patient's needs to list

Other Caregiving Skills

Can you read and understand the written information sent home by the hospital discharge planner or given to you by the home care agency, outpatient center, or other care site? This information may vary, but it might include a list of problems or diagnoses, new or changed or continuing medications, any treatments to be followed-up after discharge, any health monitoring that should occur, and other important and detailed information. There should also be a phone number and contact name with which to follow-up if you have questions. It is important to take the time to review any written information with the care manager in their presence, at the time it is presented to you—that way you will not get home and have questions because the copy of the writing was not legible or otherwise unable to be read and understood. Also, make sure you have the phone number should you have questions. This may include asking if there is an "after-hours" or on-call number to call should you have questions. This is just one example of being a prepared and proactive caregiver. There is more about this in Chapter Four: Advocacy: Your Role in Communication and Coordination.

Proactive Caregiving 101:

- Strong safety awareness
- Observation, identifying, and reporting skills
- Hands-on skills such as assisting with personal care like bathing, hair, skin, nail care, and shaving (for male patients)
- Mouth and oral care
- Catheter/tube care

- Advocacy skills
- Can follow healthcare-related instructions/direction
- Toileting care and notations related to urination (peeing) and bowel movements (BMs)
- Medication management
- Care of the bedbound person
- Assistance with activities of daily living
- Meal planning, shopping
- Meal preparation, cooking, and serving/feeding (if necessary)
- Ambulation assistance
- Assistance with walker, cane, wheelchair, lift, other assistive devices
- Laundry and assisting with dressing
- Ongoing grooming and hygiene-related activities
- Home exercise program as/if recommended by health care team
- Application/assistance with elastic or support stockings/ hose
- The use of proper safe body mechanics
- Housekeeping activities
- See a part of your role as enhancing the caregivee/loved one's quality of life every day—even if in some seemingly small way such as putting on a favorite college sports game, an old movie they like, thumbing through photo albums, or, when possible, a treat from their favorite local restaurant—or even creating a tradition where you/they go to a favorite restaurant once a week or occasionally. Consider friends, flowers, music, and/or spiritual support. These things help keep the caregivee/loved one engaged and also provide pleasure for them. Provide space and privacy for

your caregivee/loved one to spend time with family and friends.

- Identification and scheduling of supplemental assistance
- Others, as unique as your caregivee/loved one

This book is about helping you, the caregiver, find the information you need to help you best care for the caregivee/loved one. With this in mind—part of the caregiver's role is ongoing education—to help you be the best caregiver you can be. Of course readers are strongly encouraged to discuss care and related processes with the patient's care team. At the end of every chapter there are resources to help you in your education efforts. These and other resources are just that—opportunities for you to take care of yourself and improve and be knowledgeable about the needed care and what to expect for your caregivee/loved one. Remember to also ask your health care team for other resources to help you to better care for your caregivee/loved one.

Advocacy and Caregiving

The above discussion of education leads to your role as an advocate. There is a saying that "you have to know enough to know"—you can know if you read and ask and understand about the disease and caregiving activities specific to your caregivee/loved one's care. Advocacy provides you the knowledge to identify changes that should be communicated to the care team. It is for this reason that the caregiver role is so important and fundamental—you, the caregiver, become the voice of the patient when they have "no voice"—sometimes literally such as after a stroke or other health problem. An in-depth discussion about advocacy can be found in Chapter Four of this book.

These are some of the skills needed to be an effective caregiver. Many caregivers are family members while others, such as home care aides or personal care aides, are paid. One of the areas that is not listed in the above list of activities is related to financial aspects of care. This area is outside the scope of this book, but be aware that at some point, and depending on the caregivee/loved one's status, sometimes a person will no longer have the capability to "keep" the checkbook or manage their finances. Sadly, sometimes people take advantage of other's health problems, due to frailty, advanced age, and debility and/or dementia. This is called "exploitation" and should be reported to the authorities. As a caregiver, it is important that these responsibilities be clarified and decisions made in advance of the time when something happens, so that it does not have to be experienced as a "crisis." Such documents that must be planned and executed in advance so you know the person's specific wishes for effective use and planning include "power of attorney," "health care surrogate," and "advance directives."

A Health Care Home Kit

The following are only some recommended items (all available at a local pharmacy) that should be stored in a clean space in the home. Not all of these may relate to your specific needs. There may be more that your doctor, nurse, or other health care team member recommends.

- Hand sanitizer
- A thermometer
- A scale (for those who can safely stand)
- Disposable gloves
- An automated blood pressure machine (for monitoring high blood pressure, also called hypertension)
- A pulse oximeter (a medical device that monitors the oxygen saturation of a person's blood)
- A blood sugar/glucose machine (also called a glucometer; this is related to diabetes care and management)
- Medication boxes or systems that help organize caregivee's/loved one's daily/weekly medications
- Safety equipment, such as a shower chair, grab bars, etc.
- Other equipment might include a cane, a walker, a wheelchair, a bed tray, or other items as needed and ordered by your primary care provider
- Other items as directed by your care team for your caregivee/loved one's individualized care

Note: These items and others may also support the caregiver's own health—a theme you will hear throughout this handbook is the importance of maintaining your own health as well as that of your caregivee/loved one!

Summary

This chapter summarizes some of the thoughtful considerations that should be addressed about being and/or becoming a caregiver. Caregiving can be one of the most important and fulfilling roles one can assume. Not all people are or want to be caregivers. It takes a very special, empathetic, and detail-oriented person. If you wish to be/become a caregiver, this handbook can help. It is important to note that not every task that caregivers perform are listed here—caring and the caregiver's specific role is as individualized (and should be!) as the caregivee/loved one's health problems. For this reason, you are encouraged to also ask the health care team for further information, resources, instruction, and more as you care for and address your caregivee/loved ones needs. Because of the complexity of care, particularly in chronic or ongoing illness such as some cancers, diabetes, very advanced age, and other health problems, many people may be involved in the care. The next chapter will address The Care Team and Settings for Care—Health Care Today and Who's Who. This next chapter explains the health care system, who the caregiver usually interacts with, and your role to help in your caregivee's/loved one's safety, advocacy, and care plan—especially when in other health care settings such as the hospital.

Resources for You

- Aging with Dignity offers the Five Wishes resource to help guide the patient (and you!) in describing how they wish to be treated while seriously ill or unable to speak for themselves: https://www.agingwithdignity.org/five-wishes-resources.php
- The National Institute of Justice offers information on Financial Exploitation of the Elderly:http://www.nij.gov/topics/crime/elder-abuse/pages/financial-exploitation.aspx
- The National Institute on Aging offers the Elder Abuse

information page: http://www.nia.nih.gov/health/publication/elder-abuse

- The U.S. Department of Veterans Affairs offers resources for caregivers including the Preventing Medication Mishaps and Patient File Checklist documents through their Caregiver Support section: http://www.caregiver.va.gov/toolbox/toolbox_tips.asp

- USA.gov offers caregiver resources including locating tools for finding care, assisted living, home care agencies, hospices, and more at their Caregivers' Resources page: http://www.usa.gov/Citizen/Topics/Health/caregivers.shtml

- The Centers for Disease Control and Prevention offers the fact sheet Healthy Homes: Tips for Older Adults to keep the home safe for those who may be prone to falls: http://www.cdc.gov/ncbddd/disabilityandhealth/pdf/HealthyHomesOlderAdults508.pdf

- The Centers for Disease Control and Prevention also offers a focused handout on What You Can Do to Prevent Falls including a checklist for making your home safer. It includes tips like removing small throw rugs and having grab bars in the tub or showers: http://www.cdc.gov/ncipc/pub-res/toolkit/Falls_ToolKit/DesktopPDF/English/brochure_Eng_desktop.pdf

Chapter Three

The Care Team and Settings for Care—
Health Care Today and Who's Who

If there is one word to describe the health care "system" in the United States it would be complex. Because of this complexity, safety has been found to sometimes be compromised, so it is very important that you, as the caregiver, understand this big picture and the kinds of services that may be provided. Because of the complexity, it is important to note that the caregiver is the common link between specialists across care settings and transitions. In this way, they may sometimes provide a safety net to their caregivee/loved one. Safety in healthcare, in particular, is a huge issue. There was a hearing before the subcommittee on primary health and aging, 113th Congress (July 17, 2014) titled "More Than 1,000 Preventable Deaths a Day Is Too Many: The Need to Improve Patient Safety." You can view the hearing here: http://www.c-span .org/video/?320495-1/hearing-patient-safety. There is no question that work must be done to improve safety and quality— the two go hand-in-hand.

Think back to the last time you or your caregivee/loved one was in the hospital. Hopefully the hospital "stay" (this refers to his time in the hospital) went well and the reason for hospitalization, such as needing a knee replacement or having a problem after being newly diagnosed with diabetes, was addressed there, and you improved and were sent home, or your caregivee/loved one was sent home. Quality, cost, and safety are targeted areas at hospitals for improvement.

There have been safety and quality initiatives put in place by Medicare—the largest payer/insurance program which provides coverage for those over 65, those with end-stage renal disease, the disabled, and some other populations. The costs of care are outpacing available resources and sometimes the "value" of services or care, what the government pays for, is poor. As health care becomes better and more outcome-driven (meaning the quality of the care is good), consumers (patients) must assume more responsibility and have an understanding of their care and their related disease and/or health problems. This patient-centered care or "consumer focus," with increased knowledge, can only improve care and the care system. This is why we all must become very informed health care consumers—for yourself and your caregivee/loved one.

One Example—Mr. Smith

Mr. Smith was admitted for hip surgery after a fall on ice outside his home. Mr. Smith is 79 years old and has had diabetes and hypertension for many years. He is admitted to the hospital after being examined in the emergency department. While in the hospital, he develops a urinary tract infection. The rest of his hospital stay is uneventful and he is discharged to a skilled nursing facility (SNF) for three weeks of intensive rehabilitation care and then goes back to his home with a referral to a home health agency (HHA)/visiting nurse agency (VNA). The HHA nurse visits him "intermittently." The nurse reviews and manages his new medication regimen for his diabetes, high blood pressure, and a new antibiotic for his infection. In addition, a physical therapist helps Mr. Smith with his unsteady gait (or way someone walks), his balance, and an exercise program to improve his strength. An occupational therapist helps instruct Mr. Smith in activities of daily living (ADL) skills and ordering bathroom/specialized equipment. Let's review this example and Mr. Smith's course of care in some detail to see how many people he interacted with, beginning with his fall and concluding with being discharged back to home.

From the time Mr. Smith fell, he has interacted with and been cared for by many health care "providers." First it was the emergency medical services (EMS) personnel who came to his home after his neighbor called the ambulance. Then he went into the emergency room where he was cared for by a medical doctor (MD or DO), registered nurses (RNs), X-ray technicians, and others. Next, he was admitted into an inpatient area/bed in the hospital, so more new staff, nurses, aides, and laboratory personnel for blood drawing, X-ray personnel, respiratory therapists, and a new doctor, as well as other personnel, interacted with him. Mr. Smith then had surgery so there was the pre-operative service team, anesthesiologist or nurse anesthetist, the "pre-operative" services, and the operating room (OR) itself where he interfaced with surgeon(s), OR nurses, OR technicians, and possibly more OR personnel. Mr. Smith was then transferred from the OR to the recovery room (RR) where there are more doctors and nurses and other team members. After that, he went back to the postoperative care unit (which may or may not be the same inpatient unit where he was before) with more staff. He then went to a rehabilitation center and there interfaced with even more staff and therapists. In fact, while there, it was noted that he had a change in his mental status. He was confused, but had not been confused before. In this case, it is important to note that in older adult patients, a change in mental status is often the first or earliest sign of an infection. He was subsequently diagnosed with a urinary tract infection. A family member or other caregiver who "knows" Mr. Smith's usual pattern of functioning is very important for just this reason. His mental status, thus, improved after he was prescribed antibiotics. He was then finally discharged back to his home.

This is just an example and more or fewer people or levels of care could have been used across the health care setting. Either way, this is a lot of personnel and different levels and kinds of care interfacing with and caring for Mr. Smith. Such complexity—across settings of care and personnel—can create many opportunities for errors and miscommunications. Seemingly simple things, such as not calling in prescriptions for the antibiotic for his infection or his diabetes medications, could cause major problems when he returns home. These "transition points" can be where older patients may be most vulnerable for problems. Transition points occur when patients move across care settings—such as from a hospital to a rehabilitation facility, nursing home to home, or across/ between any care site or setting. This is where caregivers need to be the most informed and vigilant about their caregivee/ loved one's needs. The caregiver, for example, should know the "usual daily" medications, including doses and frequency that their caregivee/loved one takes. Medications are just one area of concern in the complexity of health care. All these areas of possible concern and miscommunication can sometimes lead to the patient being readmitted to the hospital. The topic of readmissions will be addressed later in subsequent chapters.

Safety and Quality—Important Changes

As Medicare changes to help make hospitals safer, they are also making some changes in reimbursement, or payment, to hospitals, as they realign the process and improve safety for patients. For example, because Mr. Smith acquired a urinary tract infection while in the hospital, the hospital would be financially penalized because of that. There are a list of what are called "never" events that hospitals are not generally paid for should these events happen while the patient was in the hospital. In addition to this important initiative, hospitals are also focused on helping patients remain safely at home and not coming back into the hospital. For example, the Medicare program targets hospital rates of infections from catheters in major veins and in the bladder as well as a list of potential complications from hospitalizations including blood clots, bedsores (also called pressure ulcers), and injuries, such as broken hips, from falls that happen during the hospital stay. These financial penalties are helping to drive quality improvement since hospitals are now doing much more tracking and analyses of these problems to try and minimize them. The measures include looking at infection control processes and reviewing processes related to performance improvement that may prevent problems such as falls and pressure ulcers, as well as other opportunities for performance improvement. It is hoped that these proactive approaches will be very important in reducing the number of infections and addressing other focused areas to improve patient care. Infection control is a large component of this performance improvement across all care settings, and infection control will be addressed in Chapter Seven of this book.

As you become a better, more educated consumer and caregiver for your caregivee/loved one, you may be empowered and better able to assume a more active role in preventing problems and improving healthcare outcomes. Your role in advocacy will be addressed in the next chapter, and the importance of maintaining a baseline or a care notebook or binder that you carry with you will be addressed in Chapter Five. All of this is important as more hospitals and other care settings have new safety and quality initiatives established because with safety comes quality.

A Review of Health Care Settings and Programs

The following are a list of just some of the settings where your caregivee/loved one might receive care and their definitions and descriptions. The Medicare definition of these settings will be used and then will be further explained for understanding. Some of these were settings mentioned in the above example of Mr. Smith. This list is not all inclusive—since most health care is daily and is self-care at home, this listing is only some of the most common places outside the home where your caregivee/loved one may experience care.

Assisted Living: Assisted living is for adults who need help with everyday tasks. They may need help with dressing, bathing, eating, or using the bathroom, but they don't need full-time nursing care. Some assisted living facilities are part of retirement communities. Others are near nursing homes, so a person can move easily if needs change.

Emergency Medicine: Emergency medicine specialists take care of patients with critical illnesses or injuries. Emergency departments (EDs) used to be called emergency rooms (ERs). Another type of health care center is an urgent care center and 24-hour office where you do not need an appointment; these are walk-in doctor's offices.

Home Health Care or Home Health Agency (HHA): Health care services a doctor decides through certification that you may receive in your home under a plan of care established by your doctor. Medicare only covers home health care on a limited basis and as specifically ordered/approved by your doctor.

Hospice: A special way of caring for people who have a life-threatening or life-limiting illness, such as cancer, COPD, heart failure, kidney failure, or other diseases/health problems. Hospice care involves a team-oriented approach that addresses the medical, physical, social, emotional, and spiritual needs of the patient. Hospice also provides support to the patient's family and/or caregiver(s). Hospice is a philosophy, not a setting for care, so it can be provided in any setting, including the hospital, a hospice inpatient unit, a person's home, a family member's home, or others.

Hospital Outpatient Setting: A part of a hospital where you receive outpatient services, like an emergency department, observation unit, surgery center, or pain clinic.

Inpatient Hospital Care: Treatment you get in an acute care hospital, critical access hospital, inpatient rehabilitation facility, long-term care hospital, and/or mental health care/services.

Inpatient Hospital Services: Services you get when you're admitted to a hospital, including bed and board, nursing services, diagnostic or therapeutic services, and medical or surgical services.

Nursing Home or Skilled Nursing Facility: A nursing home is a place for people who don't need to be in a hospital but can't be cared for at home. Most nursing homes have nurse's aides and skilled nurses staffed 24 hours a day. Some nursing homes are set up like a hospital. Some patients are also in nursing homes because of the need for short-term rehabilitation, such as after a stroke or orthopedic surgery. In addition, some patients are admitted from home to the facility for respite care. The staff provides medical care, as well as physical, speech and occupational therapy. There might be a nurses' station on each floor. Other nursing homes try to be more like home. They try to have a neighborhood feel. Often, they don't have a fixed day-to-day schedule, and kitchens might be open to residents. Staff members are encouraged to develop relationships with residents.

Primary Care Doctor: The doctor you see first for most health problems. He or she makes sure you get the care you need to keep you healthy. He or she also may talk with other doctors and health care providers about your care and refer you to them. In many Medicare Advantage Plans, you must see your primary care doctor before you see any other health care provider.

Skilled Nursing Facility: Skilled nursing care and rehabilitation services provided on a continuous, daily basis, in a skilled nursing facility (SNF). This may be a designated section of the nursing facility that are certified Medicare beds.

(Medicare.gov. n.d.a; Medicare.gov. n.d.b, MedlinePlus, n.d.)

Care Models: The Times They Are A-Changin'

As the cost and quality dilemma continues and decisions are made about how best to manage care and costs, other models will and are emerging. Much care is not even provided by health care professionals. In fact, some may make the case that most care is done at home and is either "self-care" or care provided by family, friends, or other (often-times unpaid) caregivers. There is also a movement toward "consumer-directed care," which is when neighbors or family members are taught to provide the person's specific care. According to the Administration for Community Living, "consumer-directed care programs encourage consumers to manage their own care. This less traditional type of Home and Community-Based Service (HCBS) program enables families to do such things as choose the type and timing of their services, hire and manage their workers, purchase supplies, make home modifications, and pay for personal care such as bathing, transporting, dressing, and other tasks" (Administration for Community Living, n.d.). Medicaid is a joint, state-administered program with support from the federal government that pays for health care for those with low incomes. Medicaid describes self-directed services as a system in which "participants, or their representatives if applicable, have decision-making authority over certain services and take direct responsibility to manage their services with the assistance of a system of available supports" (Medicaid .gov, n.d.c.).

As you become a more informed consumer, this movement toward consumer-directed care has big implications for you and your caregivee/loved one. Sometimes family members take on a very large role in care and caregiving. This might include medication administration, management and over-sight and other daily activities that perhaps your caregivee/loved one can no longer safely perform. Some hospitals teach caregivers how to provide care once back home, for example, how to change a urinary catheter, how to change a wound dressing, or other areas of responsibility. The important idea here is that more and more care will be assumed by family and/or friends as the population ages and the ranks of the gray tsunami swell. This is not only a United States-based problem—some countries in Asia have more centenarians than anywhere else in the world. All of us together must learn to give care. This overview of the health care system is just that—an overview and introduction. Readers are encouraged to read, ask questions of health care professionals, and go on tours of health care facilities—the more you know the better—and the more you can learn about care before you or your caregivee/loved one actually need it, the better.

Pulling Together Your Care Team of Support

At some point, you may be responsible for your care or your caregivee/loved one's care. This means a lot of time, complex-ity, coordination, and many other facets of care and con-cerns sometimes too numerous to list! The more you become immersed in and have some conversational understanding of the glossary and depth of caregiving and health care, the better a consumer, caregiver, or patient advocate you will be!

Consider having a list ready of the kinds of things that would be helpful for you and your caregivee/loved one for when friends, neighbors, family, spiritual community members, and/or others ask what they can do to help give you a break or help you with your caregiving responsibilities. The following are just ideas—all situations are different—but the list below may help you decide what works for you. People want to help, especially those who have been caregivers themselves. Remember that no one can do it all themselves!

- Grocery shopping
- Picking up dinner or _____ (complete the sentence)
- Running errands such as going to the post office
- Sitting with the person (presence) to allow the caregiver a break, perhaps to take a walk or a nap
- Dropping off a home cooked or ready-to-eat meal
- Helping you with home tasks such as changing beds, doing laundry, or other things
- Mowing the lawn, shoveling snow, or other yard care
- Reading to the caregivee/loved one so you can get a break

What might be offered can be as varied as the person that offers and their relationship to your family/caregivee/loved one.

Summary

The health care system is complex and no one person can know and/or do it all. Your team of support can be a varied group of family, friends, or neighbors that you may have known across time and geography. Some might be a ready ear when you need to talk or vent about situations and/or options. The axiom "no one is as smart as all of us together" is nowhere more important than in the world of healthcare and caregiving. Sometimes there is not one "right" answer—it is the one that works best for you and your caregivee/loved one and is often highly individualized. Keep in mind that "I don't know" or "I'll find out" are often honest answers to many questions. They may also tell you that there is no "right" answer to your question, especially to questions like "Will Mom get better?" The more knowledge and proactive understanding you have of health care and various programs and levels of care that you and your caregivee/loved one might need, the more effective you can be as a caregiver and consumer.

Resources for You

- What's home health care & what should I expect? from Medicare.gov explains home health care and who you can expect to be involved in care: https://www.medicare.gov/what-medicare-covers/home-health-care/home-health-care-what-is-it-what-to-expect.html
- Medicare.gov offers explanations and definitions for many terms and information concerning health care and home health: http://www.medicaid.gov/index.html
- MedlinePlus also offers definitions and explanations for many things you may encounter in the health system: http://www.nlm.nih.gov/medlineplus/
- Medicare.gov offers a booklet detailing home health care benefits including who is eligible for Medicare benefits, what services are covered, and how to find home health agencies: http://www.medicare.gov/Pubs/pdf/10969.pdf

- Medicare.gov also has a page explaining home health services: http://www.medicare.gov/coverage/home-health-services.html
- The Agency for Healthcare Research and Quality (AHRQ) provides a patient fact sheet called "Five Steps to Safer Health Care" on their website to help you and your caregivee/loved one take charge of making your own health care safer: http://www.ahrq.gov/patients-consumers/care-planning/errors/5steps/index.html
- The National Institute on Aging's AgePage offers a resource called "Hospital Hints" to prepare you for a hospital visit, including what to bring, what to leave at home, and safety tips while in the hospital: http://www.nia.nih.gov/health/publication/hospital-hints

References

Administration for Community Living (n.d.) Consumer-Directed Care. Retrieved from http://www.aoa.acl.gov/AoA_Programs/HPW/Alz_Grants/docs/Toolkit1_ConsumerDirectedCare.pdf

Medicare.gov. (n.d.a) Specialty definitions. Retrieved from http://www.medicare.gov/physiciancompare/staticpages/resources/specialtydefinitions.html

Medicare.gov. (n.d.b) Glossary. Retrieved from http://www.medicare.gov/glossary/a.html

Medicaid.gov. (n.d.c). Self Directed Services. Retrieved from http://www.medicaid.gov/Medicaid-CHIP-Program-Information/By-Topics/Delivery-Systems/Self-Directed-Services.html

MedlinePlus. (n.d.). All Health Topics. Retrieved from http://www.nlm.nih.gov/medlineplus/all_healthtopics.html

Chapter Four

Advocacy: Your Role in Communication and Coordination

Advocacy has many definitions. One Merriam-Webster definition is "a person who argues for the cause of another person in a court of law" or "a person who argues for or supports a cause or policy" (n.d.). The National Cancer Institute (NCI) defines a patient advocate as "A person who helps a patient work with others who have an effect on the patient's health, including doctors, insurance companies, employers, case managers, and lawyers. A patient advocate helps resolve issues about health care, medical bills, and job discrimination related to a patient's medical condition" (n.d.). For purposes of this chapter and clarity, advocacy will mean assuming a proactive role in which the caregiver, when appropriate and with the caregivee/loved one's permission, speaks up for or articulates and helps identify and coordinate accomplishing health care activities. In other words, the caregiver becomes the patient's voice and representative to act as an advocate for their needs.

Because of many factors, including the many kinds of clinics and specialists that may be involved in the care (such as the example of Mr. Smith having hip surgery in the previous chapter) and the ongoing theme of the complexity of care mentioned in other chapters, your caregivee/loved one needs you to be their advocate! The doctors, nurses, therapists, and others that you or your caregivee/loved one interact with cannot be expected to know EVERYTHING there is to know about one person. This, then, is your important role—for you to be knowledgeable and be able to communicate about your caregivee/loved one's needs, changes, preferences, wishes, and other related information.

Here is a real world example—a 97-year-old man lives with his adult daughter and her family. The daughter notices new large areas of bruising all up and down her father's arms. When asked, the father told his daughter that his leg was hurting (he has a long history of arthritis) and so he started taking aspirin every day. When the daughter called the doctor, the doctor directed her to stop the aspirin and recommended a topical (applied to the skin) treatment for the arthritis. This change in her father's medication regimen occurred over the phone. However, when the daughter next took her father to a scheduled doctor visit, aspirin was noted to be on the list of medications her father was taking. In this case, the daughter in her advocacy role spoke up and told the doctor about the call and the subsequent discontinuation of aspirin for her father. This shows a good example of the importance of the caregiver being the communicator and sometimes the "detail expert" to catch what might be errors in medications or other therapies and treatments. The next chapter in this book is about how to create and maintain that detailed knowledge in a care notebook or binder to help effectively communicate these important details when needed to be an effective advocate.

This example illustrates two other important points. Very few medications are without side effects—whether good or bad ones. Many think of aspirin as very safe because it can be bought "over-the-counter"—meaning without a prescription. However, like all medicines, aspirin has actions, both intended and unintended—these "actions" can be good or bad or too much or too little to be therapeutic. Many people may not realize that aspirin is a blood thinner and, therefore, like any blood thinner, it can have unintended or dangerous consequences depending on the dose, the person, other medications, and other factors.

Studies have shown that many people do not take medications as prescribed—this may be due to numerous factors, but this is important to note in any discussion of advocacy. If the doctor or nurse practitioner believes/assumes that a person is taking their medications as prescribed for a condition, such as high blood pressure or diabetes, and when examining that person at a visit notes high blood pressure is still present or that their blood sugar is high (the latter test to measure for diabetes), the clinician may then order another or more medications for these two health conditions—and this can cause further problems, such as too low blood pressure or too low blood glucose with dangerous results if the patient had not been compliant. Problems such as this can be avoided with clear communications and your advocacy role. More medications are not always better—in fact, they can sometimes lead to more side effects and problems in some cases. This specific topic will be addressed in Chapter Six: Safety in the Home: The Most Frequent Health Care Setting of Choice!

Patient and Family Representatives Have Important Roles

Many hospitals and other health care settings will welcome your level of interest and care about your caregivee/loved one. The times in health care are changing. This might be described as moving from a system where "the health care system" knows best to one where caregivers and their caregivees/loved ones are equal partners in care, care planning, goals for care, and wishes related to choices—particularly wishes related to end of life care. In fact, the Agency for Health Care Research and Quality's (AHRQ) Health Care Innovations Exchange "has identified the delivery of patient- and family-centered care (PFCC) in hospitals as a high-priority area. As defined by the Institute for Patient- and Family-Centered Care, 'patient- and family-centered care is an approach to the planning, delivery, and evaluation of health care that is grounded in mutually beneficial partnerships among health care providers, patients, and families. It redefines the relationships in health care by placing an emphasis on collaborating with people of all ages, at all levels of care, and in all health care settings. This collaboration assures that health care is responsive to an individual's priorities, preferences, and values. In patient- and family-centered care, patients and families define their "family" and determine how they will participate in care and decision-making'" (AHRQ, n.d.).

Communication Considerations—The Emergency Department

In the example above, at the doctor's office the medication change was clearly communicated and all were communicating effectively about the aspirin change to make sure that the medication list and what the patient was taking was correct and accurate. This "medication reconciliation" is one of the most important activities that one can assume/keep track of for their caregivee/loved one. The topic and definitions of medication reconciliation are addressed in depth in Chapter Six: Safety in the Home: The Most Frequent Health Care Setting of Choice! However, sometimes the communications need to be provided more urgently. This may occur when your frail or very aged caregivee/loved one or child needs to be seen or go into the emergency department or is admitted to the hospital. In these situations, it is not only important that the caregiver accompanies the patient, but is the advocate while there as well. For example, some older patients experience confusion when they are in a new or different environment. This is important to know not only for comfort reasons, but because older adults may fall when in a new or different environment. It is recommended that you stay with the person and that they be accompanied wherever they need to go—to the bathroom, to get an X-ray, or if they have to leave the room for other tests. Your calm and reassuring touch and voice can mean a great deal at this time.

And do not be afraid to speak up—if you have a question, ask it. There should be an open dialogue of communication between you and the care team of doctors and nurses. Make sure you wash your hands and those of your caregivee/loved one frequently. Consider carrying alcohol-based hand cleanser with you in your purse or otherwise on your person. Watch that doctors or nurses caring for your caregivee/loved one also wash their hands before touching. Smile and just gently remind them if this step is skipped. More often than not, there is a sink with soap and paper towels in the exam room for just this purpose. And be sure that the personnel in the exam area or the emergency room are also very aware of infections. Tell them if you or your caregivee/loved one has been sick with a cold, was diagnosed with or has symptoms of influenza, has diarrhea, and/or has been taking antibiotics.

The change in environment mentioned above can cause your caregivee/loved one to exhibit either confusion or more confusion than usual. They may also become disoriented as to the day, place, or other usually known information. There can be other causes of dementia symptoms. Because of this, a thorough evaluation and diagnostic work-up should be done before there is a diagnosis of dementia. For example, normal pressure hydrocephalus (NPH) can also cause dementia and the dementia from NPH is potentially reversible. Depression, psychosis, vitamin deficiency, and other medical problems should also be investigated. This "befuddlement" or new mental confusion can be a result of the change in environment and other factors, such as an acute infection. This is particularly true of urinary tract infections in older adults. It can get even more complex and troubling when medications are given as part of the treatment. For these and other reasons, emergency departments (EDs) and other health care settings that the person does not know can be unsettling and problematic. Try to help with your caregivee/loved one's comfort by asking for warm towels (sometimes health care settings can be very cold, especially to the very old who feel cold more generally). If your caregivee/loved one attempts to stand, be there to help and have them use the handrails that may be in the healthcare setting for safety. Your holding on to your caregivee/loved one or walking on their other side is also a good thing. The bathroom toilet can also be an opportunity for a fall—ask for a bedside commode or a bedpan to be brought into the room if that seems safer. Remember that you are the expert on your caregivee/loved one's situation—and your number one priority is to get them back home safely. Some emergency rooms and other health systems are creating areas specifically designed for older patients and their unique safety needs. This makes sense given the growing number and demographics of the aging population! Similarly, pediatric emergency departments at pediatric hospitals are designed around children and their specialized care needs. The caregivers, oftentimes the parents, are the experts in their children and the child's needs.

When you are ready to leave the care setting, make sure that you understand what the diagnoses or problem was and that you have written and legible instructions about what you are to do for your caregivee/loved one until they next see their regular primary doctor, nurse practitioner, or whomever they are referred to for follow-up care and when that next appointment is. It is important for continuity of care reasons that you ask that the discharge summary be faxed or emailed to your caregivee/loved one's primary care provider and that you also received a copy to take to your next primary care provider appointment in case it did not arrive. If antibiotics or another new medication was mentioned or started (meaning a dose was given) while there, make sure that you have the written prescription in hand when you leave the ED (also ask if any medications should be stopped). It is very important that your caregivee/loved one's primary physician know the names of all the physicians involved in their care and the pharmacies that are providing medications. If the prescription is filled at a pharmacy not normally used, bring your medication list for the pharmacist to check for interactions. Even better, ask that the medication be "called in" by the ED doctor to your local pharmacy. This is a good idea since that local pharmacy may know all the medications that your caregivee/loved one is taking. In this way, the pharmacist can check for any drug interactions or other considerations between the medications your patient is already on and this new medication. Also ask who you should call—both a name and a number—should you have questions once back home. Ask what number to call after regular hours and, if necessary, how their "on-call" system works.

Facts About Falls

It was mentioned above about changes in environment for your caregivee/loved one in different settings. Falls are a concern whenever your caregivee/loved one is changing settings or environments, especially in the ED. According to the AHRQ between 700,000 and 1 million patients experience a fall in U.S. hospitals every year (2013) and between 20–30% of all falls result in moderate to severe injury (Centers for Disease Control and Prevention, 2014). Falls and their prevention are a very complex patient safety issue as many factors are associated with falls. Some of these factors include age, a history of falls and associated fear of falling, frailty, chronic conditions, weak muscles, medications, dementia, urinary frequency, trouble walking, a history of fainting or seizures, a drop in blood pressure upon standing (called orthostatic hypotension), decreased sensation, use of assistive devices such as walkers or canes, and many other factors. For this reason, when your caregivee/loved one is admitted to a hospital, home health agency, or other setting, there may be a fall "risk assessment" completed. Sometimes an older adult might not see their own frailty. This is where your advocacy and communication skills as a caregiver are very important. And some older people do not want others to even know they have fallen. For these reasons, it is very important that an accurate fall-risk assessment and history be completed. This information needs to be reviewed on an ongoing basis and written into the person's specific plan of care for caution and safety reasons. Falls are discussed in depth in Chapter Six: Safety in the Home: The Most Frequent Health Care Setting of Choice!

Communication Considerations—In the Hospital and Beyond

Caregivers need to stay vigilant when your caregivee/loved one is in the hospital. Like the ED, it is a change in the environment and so a risk area for falls or other unwanted events. Once admitted to the hospital, and especially after first being in the ED, your caregivee/loved one may be very tired. Being tired or exhausted may also contribute to falls. The older adult may be confused or disoriented and not be able to use the "call light." It may be that the bed is "high" and the older adult may not be able to use the mechanism to lower it before getting out of bed. Always encourage them to sit on the side of the bed and "dangle" their feet and sit upright for a few minutes before attempting to stand. Some older people get what is called "orthostatic hypotension," orthostatic meaning a change in position, which causes hypotension, otherwise called a drop in blood pressure. This orthostatic hypotension may cause the person to fall. Sitting on the bedside for a few minutes before standing helps the blood get to where it needs to be and, therefore, may help decrease such incidents and perhaps prevent a fall. The topics of falls are a huge concern to all involved, so this is another important role for the advocate. Falls are a complex and multifactorial issue, so prevention is key when possible!

Hopefully your caregivee/loved one has an advanced directive and has communicated and put in writing what they want and do not want related to end of life care and care planning. Not only should the issues be discussed prior to arriving in the hospital, but the issues also need to be revisited/updated on an on-going basis. This discussion or conversation should be already accomplished (hopefully) long before the time you reach the hospital, but just in case it has not yet been taken care of, readers might wish to visit the website www.fivewishes.org.

Some family members take turns staying with the caregivee/loved one while they are in the hospital. Staying overnight can be reassuring, especially to the caregivee/loved one, and many family members do this—it should go without saying, though, that you and any visitors should not be loud, on a cell phone, and/or otherwise disruptive in any way. In this way, they are not alone and the caregiver can help them stay oriented by reminding the person that they are in the hospital and why and can call for help if needed. Bedside call lights can be difficult for older persons, especially if they have any confusion, and they may forget to use the call light at all. Generally advocate and be their voice.

Here is an example that shows the importance of your presence and just being there. You may be there to ask "why and what is it for?" when there is a new medication to be given. If the doctor did not mention a new medication, you have the right to question what the medication is and if the doctor prescribed it. It is okay to say you want to talk with the doctor first—before it is given—especially since it is in this way that medication errors are sometimes avoided. You should expect to be kept updated of what the plan is for your caregivee/loved one. For example, if a new medication or treatment is added that you were not aware of, ask to speak to the staff and/or see the doctor.

Like in the ED, hand hygiene and hand washing is critically important—did hospital team members wash their hands? If you are not sure, do not be afraid to ask!

Note that it is very important that caregivers and family members not be demanding or rude to the healthcare team. This is truly a team effort when it works. It is important to remember that nurses, doctors, and patient care technicians (PCTs) are working with many patients and while being a good advocate, also be mindful of their time and other responsibilities. If you have a lot of non-urgent questions, consider asking them to come back at a convenient time to help better address your questions and allow them to complete their other tasks. Write down your questions so that when they do return, it is an organized process and you get all your questions answered.

Remember that NO ONE can know it all, so speak up and ask when you do not understand something! It is always better to ask than assume in health care! You can say no (patients have rights) and ask to speak to the doctor or the charge nurse if you are ever unsure or uncomfortable.

Discharge should not be a surprise. People do not stay in the hospital long, but there needs to be communication about the plan for discharge. You should know when to expect discharge and what to expect after it—when there will be follow-up visits; medications to be prescribed and picked up; other services being provided, such as home health or therapy; etc.

Like at home, you might want to keep a log of how your caregivee/loved one is doing. It is recommended that you also write down any questions or thoughts you wish to discuss with the doctors or care team for the next doctor or nurse visit. Because of the complexity of health care, it can be easy to forget a question. In this way, you are ready with your notes and questions and won't forget an important point. Ask about any test results, too—what they are, what will they tell us about the condition, and, as important, what is the plan if/when something is found? If you will be travelling to another area, you might consider requesting copies of medical test results or coordinating the transfer of records to the new physician.

Here is another example. The doctor wants to do a colonoscopy for a 95-year-old woman who had a history of colon cancer. In this case, the woman had no problems and it was called a follow-up screening. This woman wanted no surgery or treatment at this point in her life even if something had been found so she declined this unnecessary procedure. You can say no at any time and sometimes common sense will tell you what is right.

Like the ED, there should be clear and legible information provided about your caregivee's/loved one's care plan for discharge. Make sure you understand what is to happen next before you leave.

Sometimes the caregivee/loved one may be discharged from the hospital to a new environment, such as an assisted living center, or they may be referred to home health or hospice. It is okay to ask questions about this when you need it. The hospital has discharge planners and social workers just for this reason. They are usually the experts on local facilities and resources in the community. They may also be able to tell you about support groups, additional support, other caregivers, or other resources as you identify support you need for your caregivee/loved one.

Summary

This chapter defines advocacy and its importance in the role of being an active, engaged, and knowledgeable caregiver. These skills are particularly important when your caregivee/ loved one is in the hospital or other new care setting. This chapter emphasizes that there are no dumb questions. Your role is to help protect your caregivee/loved one and perhaps prevent problems.

Resources for You

- The Joint Commission sponsored a program based on Institute of Medicine (IOM) findings that encourages advocacy to help avoid medical errors: http://www.jointcommission .org/assets/1/6/speakup.pdf
- The National Institute on Aging offers a booklet called Long-Distance Caregiving: Getting Started that discusses how you can play a role even if you do not live close to the person needing care: http://www.nia.nih.gov/health/ publication/long-distance-caregiving-getting-started
- The National Institute on Aging also offers a booklet on

Medicines: Use Them Safely to help you understand what to ask the doctor and what to ask the pharmacist when you or your caregivee/loved one is prescribed a medicine: http://www.nia.nih.gov/health/publication/medicines

References

Agency for Healthcare Research and Quality (AHRQ). (2013). "Preventing Falls in Hospitals A Toolkit for Improving Quality of Care" Retrieved from http://www.ahrq.gov/professionals/systems/hospital/fallpxtoolkit/fallpxtoolkit.pdf

Agency for Healthcare Research and Quality (AHRQ). (n.d.). "Advancing the Practice of Patient- and Family-Centered Care in Hospitals" Retrieved from https://innovations.ahrq.gov/node/8269

Centers for Disease Control and Prevention (CDC). (2014). "Costs of Falls Among Older Adults" Retrieved from http://www.cdc.gov/HomeandRecreationalSafety/Falls/fallcost.html

Merriam-Webster.com. (n.d.). "advocate." Retrieved from http://www.merriam-webster.com/dictionary/advocate

National Cancer Institute (NCI). (n.d.). "patient advocate." Retrieved from http://www.cancer.gov/dictionary?cdrid=44534

Chapter Five

Creating and Maintaining a Care Notebook or Binder (Or Take This with You to the Doctor, Nurse, or Hospital!)

The prior chapter emphasized the importance of clear and ongoing communications between you, the caregiver, as a consumer of health care and the members of the health care team. Mutual respect, listening skills, and validation of what was said and/or what was understood are important parts of this ongoing communications and relationship. This chapter presents a format or easy method of how to organize and present this important and, sometimes, crucial information to those involved across the "care continuum." This "care continuum" refers to all the varying levels and types of care and providers who may care for you and/or your caregivee. This includes the hospital; a skilled nursing facility; a nursing home; a rehabilitation center; an assisted living facility; out-patient areas, including the doctor's office; and home.

Although one of the intents of the notebook is a chronologic history of your caregivee/loved one's healthcare information, it may also be very helpful when a loved one has confusion. For example, keeping a care notebook may have an area where family members can sign in and leave notes for their loved one who has confusion. This allows the confused person to access some information about when their family visits. This can help ease distress about the "family never visiting." This can help relieve some degree of angst and anxiety about the lack of caring from friends and family.

Creating a Care Notebook or Binder for Communication

Consider creating what can be called a "care notebook" or binder where anything health-related is housed and noted. This could include appointments, treatments, and laboratory values/results—the one place where health information is kept and noted. Sections of the care book/binder could be the calendar of scheduled visits/appointments, laboratory tests, X-rays, and other findings and result information. You could also have pages with your own notes that might explain why the doctor saw your caregivee/loved one that day (such as a scheduled visit or they got sick and needed to be seen for a specific problem), if they were started on a new medication, and, as important, what the new medication is for or what it is treating specifically.

There is no question that it can be very hard to keep all this information straight—and no one should rely on memory given the complexity of care from both safety and quality perspectives. The care notebook or binder is one way to help you do just that! Include "patient identifiers," such as a picture, a driver's license, health insurance card (a copy), or other identification. Also include other very important health-related documents including an end-of life section that addresses end-of-life wishes and/or any signed documents, such as a "Do Not Resuscitate" (DNR) form or advanced directive. This information might be filed in the front of the binder with the most updated medication list for ease of retrieval. Such information is fundamental to safety because care providers need to be sure of and verify the identity of the patient—and that the "right person" gets the right medications and treatments. In fact, if your caregivee/loved one is in the hospital, they will be asked innumerable times for their name and date of birth.

You should also list all medications—what the medication is for, allergies, discontinued and start dates, their dose, route (how they are taken, i.e., by mouth, as eye drops, etc.), indication (since many medications are used for multiple reasons), how often (how many times a day they are to be taken), with or without food, and any other relevant information. This also includes medications that you take as needed or what is called "PRN." It can also be important to note if medications have been changed or doses have been changed or stopped. This should include over-the-counter medications as well as any herbs or other "remedies," not just prescription medications. Your doctor and pharmacist should have a complete list and everyone should use this list and ensure that is correct, accurate, and up-to-date at all times. This is called "medication reconciliation" and this process of checking for accuracy is very important for safety and quality reasons. That is why when one goes to the doctor or the emergency department the providers ask about medications. For safety, it is essential that the caregiver keep a list in their wallet or purse for unexpected situations that lists all the medications referenced above in one place.

There should be a calendar to keep track of doctor and other care-related visits or care, including hospitalizations, emergency department visits, or others. And, just as important, what happened at those visits or care encounters. Part of the high cost of health care occurs when tests are repeated because results cannot be located. In addition to being expensive, this is also wasteful. You may have your caregivee/loved one sign a privacy release so that you can both access and receive copies of any X-rays, blood or urine tests, etc. In this way, you have a record of them and they are housed in one place—your care notebook or binder.

A Visual Model: You and Your Caregivee/ Loved One as the Hub of the Wheel!

Depending on your caregivee/loved one's health problems, there may be various types of doctors and others involved in their care. This can contribute to miscommunications because of the complexity of health problems and the number of people involved. The caregiver—you—can be the one person who knows all the disparate or different facets of care. Think of your caregivee and yourself as the center of a circle, or the hub. Then imagine spokes or lines coming out from around the center. For example, a person with bladder cancer and diabetes may be cared for by an oncologist (a cancer doctor), a urologist (a specialist in urinary care for prostate and perhaps bladder problems), an endocrinologist (a specialist in endocrine problems of which diabetes is the most common) and perhaps others if the person is also getting radiation or other specialized treatments for the cancer. In addition, they may also be seeing an internist or family practice physician or a nurse practitioner or a physician's assistant for primary care for conditions such as depression or anxiety. They may also be seeing an opthomologist (for their eyes), a dentist, a chiropractor, or other providers.

Practically, what this means is that each specialist/office is only getting a small slice or snapshot of the big circle/picture. And the big picture is the complexity of your caregivee as a person and their related and unique health challenges. "Related" because as you may have learned from the "Care Sections" of this book that many conditions are interrelated (such as diabetes and heart problems and depression) and treatments or other health care problems may have "side" effects that negatively impact how the patient "feels" or functions "day to day." An example could be that the patient received chemotherapy and this caused them to be more susceptible to infections. Or a patient or person might have pain and some of the medications used to treat the pain may make the person feel "foggy" or not clear in their thinking and/or very constipated. Many conditions and treatments contribute to the complexity of care and the resolution of health problems.

If you know and can "see" the big picture and who all the players are that are involved in care, sometimes only you have the entire comprehensive "view" of your caregivee's unique care needs and specific problems. This care notebook will be a "holistic" (meaning provide an entire view) collection of their care. It is a compilation of all care, so the binder or notebook will grow in size each time you go to the doctor, change a treatment, or get new medications. Consider getting three ring binders, a hole puncher, and plan to begin on a certain date. If your caregivee is fairly stable, you might make it a goal to organize the material and start on the first day of the next month (such as March 1 if it is February). The date does not matter as much as the data!

Begin by filing things chronologically and in order (such as

January, February, etc. to be able to easily access and identify needed information. An example could be that your caregivee had never been known to be allergic to any medications, but when they were started on a new anti-inflammatory medication for pain, they developed symptoms consistent with an allergy and it was stopped after you, as the caregiver, called the doctor and told them about the problem. This important information—what the name of the drug is, both brand and generic names if known—should be documented and what the specific allergic reaction/problems identified were. Any allergies, whether new or already known, should be noted in the care notebook/binder. In addition, consider obtaining bright colored labels at the office supply store and listing the allergies your caregivee has. Make "stickers" out of the bright colored labels and place them outside on your binder—either the cover or the spine. In this way, when speaking with any member of the care team you can—at a glance at the colored sticker—know what your caregivee is allergic to and quickly communicate that information. Make sure information about the pharmacy/pharmacist that you work with is also included in your binder, preferably filed at the beginning of the medication section.

Here is another example. You called the doctor about your caregivee with a urinary catheter because the urine is more dark than usual and the urine "smells" (and you also know that your caregivee/loved one has a history of urinary tract infections). In this example, someone from the doctor's office calls you back (usually not a nurse anymore, it may be a medical technician or an administrative assistant; it is ok to ask to whom you are speaking) and says they are calling in a prescription for penicillin. Getting to know the names and the people who work with your doctor's office team can be very helpful in care coordination and effective communication. In this example, another doctor is covering for your caregivee/loved one's primary physician and so that doctor may not know about any allergies your caregivee/loved one has—but, at a glance, you know that your caregivee cannot take that specific medication because you have listed penicillin on the care sticker on the outside of the care notebook. Such fundamental processes can sometimes help make the difference between a miscommunication and an error—the goal here is to prevent a problem! Safety and quality must be the watchwords of effective and knowledgeable caregivers. There are no secrets. The more educated the caregiver and all of us can be about health care (as opposed to sick care!), the better we will be. So try and read all you can about your and your caregivee/loved one's health problems.

And another safety tip—do not limit the allergies that you track to medications. There might also be allergies to such things as latex, iodine and foods (such as shellfish, peanuts, etc.) as well as other substances. All of these are also important to note as medications may have some of these products in them and latex is often in gloves and other medical supplies.

One more thing about medications—since you are the person who knows ALL the medications and over-the-counter items, vitamins, etc., that your caregivee/loved takes, consider working with or using one pharmacy (only) when possible. This way, one pharmacy and its pharmacists know what your caregivee is on and they can check for any interactions or other possible medication-related problems—sometimes before they occur. A good local pharmacy and pharmacist can make all the difference, plus they are the expert on medications and easily accessible and understandable when one has questions. Ask the pharmacist for a printout of all your medications and all drug-drug interactions and side effect information available. Do not hesitate to ask them these questions—there are no dumb questions in health care, only the questions that do not get asked. No one can know it all so when in doubt—ask, ask, ask!

Another idea for consideration, depending on the amount of care, providers, complexity, and other factors, is the possibility of hiring a care manager. A care manager can coordinate your caregivee/loved one's care and they specialize in this complexity. Be aware that some private insurance companies have case or care management programs for certain diagnoses, such as asthma, heart failure, and others.

Care managers know resources and health systems and their foibles. Geriatric care managers may be nurses or social workers. Visit http://www.aginglifecare.org to locate care managers near you. They often accompany people to doctor appointments and provide consistent coordination across care sites and provider types. They can reconcile the patient's medications, locate needed resources, and much more, all based on a comprehensive assessment.

7 Tips for Making Your Doctor or Nurse Practitioner Visits More Productive—Bring Your Care Notebook with You!

The following tips in this section are to help you and your caregivee/loved one have more effective visits with your primary care provider.

1. Write down any questions in advance of your caregivee/ loved one's office visit. This especially includes why you called and made the appointment—such as "I have noticed a change in the caregivee/loved one's balance" or "my caregivee/loved one fell twice in the last month or has some new pain." Bring all that with you as the office will need to update your caregivee/loved one information and this helps assure its accuracy. You may also be asked to present a picture identification card.

2. Come about 15 minutes ahead of time if possible. There will be HIPAA (privacy) forms, consent forms, or other information to complete. In this way, you may be calmer and more organized so you can better concentrate on your visit.

3. Hygiene is very important. You want the doctor or NP to take the time needed to assess and critically think to determine the best course of action(s) for you. This does not mean pouring on a gallon of after shave or perfume (actually, that may negatively impact others in the waiting area). It does mean shaving, good oral hygiene, and a bath or shower prior to the appointment. Having worked in emergency departments and other areas in hospitals, I know this sounds fundamental, but you would be shocked! When in doubt, put yourself in the role of the provider who must get very close and personal in their duties! And since we are on the subject of hygiene—hand hygiene comes to mind! Wash your and your caregivee's/loved one's hands before the visit and after the visit. And it is okay to watch and make sure that all who touch you and/or your caregivee/loved one also perform hand hygiene—this may be the doctor, nurses, the NP, or any aides or assistants.

4. Have and use glasses, teeth, hearing aids, and/or other

devices that help you or caregivee/loved one! This may include a cane, a walker, or a splint. It is important that the NP or the doctor see your caregivee/loved one as you function at home and in the community—they are just getting a small "snapshot" of you both. This helps show how your caregivee/loved one is functionally, which is very important to their assessment and care.

5. Carry that list of questions that you wrote down in #1 and add to it any specific changes you have noted since your last office visit/encounter. This may include changes with any body system or other things you notice or your caregivee/loved one reports. I sometimes have older friends who say "I think this is old age"—many things are not "old age" and pain and many other symptoms or changes should not be so readily attributed to this. Also, if this is a doctor or NP who does not know your specific circumstances (such as you are vacationing and get some kind of cold or a bug) tell them how your caregivee/loved one usually is—their usual activity level, etc. This is the reason you are here for this visit so try and be as clear as you can in communicating what is happening that brought your caregivee/loved one to the office visit and why it is not normal for them. It is also always good to be proactive. If you are planning an international or other big trip or significant travel, tell the doctor or NP. Similarly, if you or your caregivee/loved one were on vacation and came home sick, tell them this information including where you traveled to and from. More information and history is better when it comes to telling a complete health story.

6. Ask for any refills for prescriptions while you are there at the office. This is the time to coordinate all these related

activities. And, if your pharmacy has changed, also communicate that information to the provider (they may ask for the address and phone number of the pharmacy you use). Also have this information with you and handy if possible.

7. Be a partner in your and your caregivee's/loved one's health. Listen to the instructions and adhere to the medication or other regimen that the doctor or NP provides. Make any follow-up appointments and follow the provider's advice. This may include such things as to cut down on salt, increase your physical activity, and others. Simply put, the doctor or NP may see you or your caregivee/loved one a few times a year, but your health care is what you do every day—it includes choices we make in eating/nutrition, exercising, sleep habits, lifestyle, and many others. Most of us can make more healthful choices in our everyday lives. This is what health truly is—not the absence of illness or disease. We all have very important roles to play in our health. The doctor or NP visit is one important component of that health journey!

Summary

A care binder or notebook is one way to track and organize the information that is important to providing continuity of care across care settings and as a tool to help communication and coordination about your caregivee/loved one's needs and health problems. The following pages provide links to some sample forms that you may wish to use or recreate to help you keep track of some of this information. They include medication forms, forms for tracking blood pressures, blood sugars, and other tests and findings. Bringing this care note-book into the doctor, nurse, or other health care setting will help your caregivee/loved one get better care because you are an active part of the care planning team.

Tools, Forms, and Resources for You

- The U.S. Department of Veterans Affairs offers resources on their website including checklists like the Patient File Checklist to help you choose what to put in your binder: http://www.caregiver.va.gov/toolbox/index.asp
- For an example of an adult medical history questionnaire, the MD Anderson Cancer Center offers a pdf of one on their site. This can help you get an idea of what information you may need to have ready when you fill out paperwork at the doctor's office: https://my.mdanderson.org/forms/PHDB.pdf
- MIT also offers a similar form for children: https://medical.mit.edu/pdf/pedshistory.pdf
- The Centers for Disease Control and Prevention (CDC) offer an immunization and development milestone chart if your caregivee/loved one is young: http://www.cdc.gov/vaccines/parents/downloads/milestones-tracker.pdf
- The American Heart Association offers a blood pressure tracking form: https://www.heart.org/idc/groups/heart-public/@wcm/@hcm/documents/downloadable/ucm_305157.pdf
- The American Diabetes website offers a form to keep track of blood glucose levels: http://professional.diabetes.org/

admin/UserFiles/file/Reducing%20Cardiometabolic%20
Risk_%20Patient%20Education%20Toolkit/English/
ADA%20CMR%20Toolkit_29BloodGlucose.pdf

- The University of Michigan's health system has an incontinence log available: http://www.uofmhealth.org/sites/
default/files/healthwise/media/pdf/hw/form_aa137606.pdf
- The Louisiana Department of Health and Hospitals offers a
bowel movement log for tracking changes in bowel habits,
which could be especially helpful if your caregivee/loved
one is on pain medication: http://dhh.louisiana.gov/assets/
docs/OCDD/publications/bowellog.pdf
- The United Mitochondrial Disease Foundation offers sample forms including a medication administration log and a
hospitalization and surgery log: http://www.umdf.org/atf/
cf/%7B858ACD34-ECC3-472A-8794-39B92E103561%7D/8_
FORM_TITLE_PAGE&FORMS.PDF
- SafeMedication offers a medicine list for you to fill in to
keep track of the medications you are on as well as things
like allergies you may have and emergency contact information: http://www.safemedication.com/safemed/My
MedicineList/MyMedicineList_1.aspx
- The U.S. Food and Drug Administration (FDA) has a "My
Medicine Record" resource to help you track your med-
ications, including information about how many times a
day it is taken and what it looks like: http://www.fda.gov/
downloads/AboutFDA/ReportsManualsForms/Forms/
UCM095018.pdf
- AARP offers a medication record for you to fill out in
Spanish: http://assets.aarp.org/www.aarp.org_/articles/
health/docs/spanish_personal_med_record.pdf
- The National Institutes of Health have an article from June

2015 about "Talking With Your Doctor: Making the Most of Your Appointment" in their monthly newsletter, News in Health: http://newsinhealth.nih.gov/issue/jun2015/feature2

References

National Heart, Lung, and Blood Institute. (n.d.) High Blood Pressure Detection. Retrieved from https://www.nhlbi.nih.gov/hbp/detect/detect.htm

Chapter Six

Safety in the Home: The Most Frequent Health Care Setting of Choice!

In Chapter Three, we discussed quality and safety in terms of the hospital and other care settings—other than the home. This chapter focuses, instead, on quality and safety in the home setting. Safety in the home is crucial. We need to start viewing healthcare with home as the "hub" and all other spokes originating from this center of the wheel. The fundamentals of health and health habits are started, maintained, and housed there! The home is central to health care since it is the main environment where health is supported, or not, by daily actions. Simply put, people do not live in hospitals—it is to the home where people are discharged back to and where healthcare must be supported, provided, and enhanced. Because most caregiving is provided at home, this chapter addresses the safety and quality issues specific to the home setting. I believe that home will be the future hub of health care, and safety and quality are the pivotal variables that can help make that vision work!

When people are surveyed and asked where they would like to receive care and, if at the end of life, die, they usually answer "home." AARP (formerly known as the American Association of Retired Persons) found that 89% of Americans wanted to stay in their current home as long as they could

(2010). There truly is no place like home! Sadly, many people who wish to remain at home do not. AARP also found that many older adults constantly fear having to go into a nursing home (2010).

This chapter is all about keeping your caregivee/loved one at home when possible and safe to do so. This entire book, and this chapter specifically, is crafted to help you and your caregivee/loved one remain at home—with safety in mind. Because of the many facets and factors that may impact safety in the home environment, this chapter is framed around the word "H-O-M-E" as a way to organize all these important components. H stands for the House/Home, O stands for Objective (View), M stands for Medication-Related Safety, and E stands for the Environment of the home. In this way, some of the most important problems related to safety will be addressed to help you and your caregivee/loved one remain safe and at home.

H—The House/Home Environment

Every home is different and we all live in different ways. This includes such choices as how "clean" the house is (what is good for some people others consider dirty or not-so-clean), how many pets we might have—and where they are allowed or not allowed—and numerous other factors that, together, contribute to how we live in a house. And the actual house varies too! It may be a "split-level" with stairs, a one level ranch, or a condo with an elevator. It is safe to say that a house is as unique as its owner(s).

What a house "looks like" and how the layout flows is usually not a problem—until the caregivee/loved one has a health problem that becomes an impediment to staying in the home. Here is an example: A 79-year-old man falls off a ladder at his home (that choice is a discussion for another day!) and he comes home after surgery with a cast on his leg and his arm. His wife and he have a master bedroom that is upstairs. This is an older home and all the bathrooms are upstairs so this becomes a dilemma when it is time for him to be discharged from the hospital and go home. A hospital bed is delivered and the only place it will fit is wedged into the dining room. A commode chair is a chair that looks like a toilet that is mobile and is used in place of being able to get to a bathroom, is also delivered by the home medical equipment company (sometimes called a durable medical equipment company, or HME or DME). All these items are now located in their downstairs "living" space. To make things worse, the wheelchair that was also delivered cannot fit through the doorways of the home. Such supports and conveniences can seem like an "easy" fix—but they are not. Such arrangements have privacy, logistic, and other implications. This is why many new homes are being built with wider door frame widths, tile instead of carpet, no thresholds, master suites on the first floor, or even no stairs. This is so that floors are one level should someone perhaps need to use a wheelchair or a walker. As we all age, thoughtful consideration must be given to the home structure that allows people to truly "age in place." Another phrase that is frequently used and also ties into safety is "home modification." Simply put, these are changes or modifications made to adapt one's living space to meet the needs of an aging population or for those with other physical limitations so that they can continue to comfortably and safely live in their home. Such modifications can vary and may include making spaces bigger, adding an elevator or a chair lift, adding a wheelchair ramp, having a bedroom and bathroom downstairs, adding handrails to stairs, adding grab bars in the bathroom, and more. The time to think about this is before these safety accommodations are needed. Consider a home evaluation prior to discharge from the hospital or skilled nursing facility. In addition, there may be cost issues for some of the adaptations needed to adapt the home to the caregivee/loved one.

O—Objective (View)

It is natural that when we have lived somewhere for a while, we can sometimes no longer "see" things. Many items or furnishings and their placement become "background" to busy, daily living. Now, try to objectively walk into your house and look around and try to pretend that you have never "seen" it before. Think back to the example of the man in the above section who came back home after a fall. How would you experience this same situation? Would the space functionally work for you with the hospital bed, commode, and wheelchair, and would you be able to remain downstairs? Would privacy be an issue? This objective view is also very important for you, the caregiver, should you also seek to age in place (which simply means staying at home as you age).

In Chapter Two, there was a list of considerations about the space where the caregivee/loved one would be cared for and questions related to its adequacy and safety. This discussion is more related to the safety of the actual home space with the knowledge of the most common safety problems that impact older adults and children at home. The first immediate topic is fire safety. Now that you have walked around and looked at your space with those "new eyes"—what did you see and notice specifically? From a safety perspective, always try to consider prevention and how to minimize dangers in that environment. The best prevention starts with a safety check in each room of your home. Are there working smoke alarms and carbon monoxide detectors? Are the batteries working? Are there easy ways to exit the house should there be a fire? If you have a wood stove or chimney, has the flue been professionally cleaned recently? Can your caregivee/loved one be carried out? What is the specific plan should there be a fire or other reason for evacuation? Consider putting flashlights beside your beds for power outages and safety. Simply put, what is/are the escape route(s) and plan? Such questions are particularly important if the caregivee/loved one is "bedbound" or uses life-sustaining technology at home, such as oxygen or a ventilator.

Other fundamentals to consider, assess, and observe are the furniture and furnishings. For one example, how difficult (or easy) is it for an older adult at home to get up out of a chair? Adjusting the height of the seat and chair arms can help with this problem. Chairs that are (too) low and without arms can present a problem for older adults who have poor strength, balance, and/or are frail when they try to get out of a chair. Sofas can also be a problem for the same reasons. Throw rugs and extension cords present hazards that are usually easily removed. Consider purchasing furniture risers to improve height and safety.

Take a good look at the bathroom(s). It has been said that bathrooms are the most dangerous rooms in a house. (Kitchens are also dangerous because of fire risks, which is discussed later in this chapter.) There are a lot of hard surfaces in bathrooms, such as porcelain toilets, tubs, sinks, and hard floors made of tile or wood. Hot water can also be dangerous and should be checked for temperature. Consider a bathing or shower chair, a handheld shower head to help the caregiver when assisting the caregivee/loved one in the shower, and no-slip floors on the shower floor and in the bathroom generally and grab bars in the shower and around the toilet. Remember to turn on a light or a night light in the bathroom and bedroom of the caregivee/loved one before it gets dark as balance can be impacted by poor or no light and they could trip on something they cannot see because it is dark. Remove all bath mats when not in use, especially if the caregivee/love one uses an assistive device, such as a walker, cane, or wheelchair.

The Kitchen—Why It Can Be a Dangerous Place

Kitchens are considered by many as the "heart" of the home. Sadly, cooking fires are the number one cause of home fires in America according to the U.S. Fire Administration (USFA) (2012). Older adults, age 65 and older, are "more than twice as likely to die in fires than the Nation's population as a whole" (2012). Scalding and burn injuries often occur because older adults may have decreased vision, balance, and other problems and frailties that can contribute to these injuries. If the caregivee/loved one has worked in the same kitchen for many years, it can be understood that they do not "see" the pitfalls or any dangers in their space. Especially if there is an open flame, such as a gas stove, it is important to be particularly careful. Loose-fitting clothes or bathrobes with belts or other loose items should not be worn while cooking or in the kitchen because they can easily ignite. The same can be said for using hand towels to hold hot pots or pans instead of mittens or potholders. Tight clothes should be worn around the open flame of a gas stove. Obviously this information also applies to children. Also, never leave the stove or a toaster unattended. The caregiver must be aware at all times about fire safety, especially kitchen fire safety, and its prevention.

Oxygen Considerations and Safety

Your caregivee/loved one may be on oxygen therapy; this would be ordered by the physician, with specific orders or usage parameters, like any other treatment. The use of oxygen in the home has serious safety and other implications. In one report, there were an average of 1,190 burn patients seen every year in an emergency department caused by ignitions (meaning caught on fire) associated with the use of home medical oxygen (National Fire Protection Association, 2008). Most of these were facial burns (National Fire Protection Association, 2008).

Here are just some of the rules related to the use of home medical oxygen. First, there can be NO SMOKING! There can also never be an open flame or a candle in the room. Check that you have working smoke alarms. There should be "no smoking" and other signage that alert those coming into the home that there is oxygen in use and, thus, no smoking! Do not use a wood stove or a match or any other kind of open flame when oxygen is in use. This also includes cigarettes, candles, and gas stoves. Oxygen creates an environment where any fire that might start burns faster and hotter. Do not use petroleum-based products for those on oxygen.

If your caregivee/loved one is on oxygen, ask your supplier for signs and pamphlets with more specific safety information. The HME or DME company may have respiratory therapist professionals who are the experts about oxygen therapy and its safe use at home.

M—Medication-Related Safety

Medication errors are the most frequent type of medical error across the health care system (Garrouste-Orgeas, 2012). Medications and medicines are one of the largest reasons that older adults come to the emergency department (ED) and sometimes into the hospital (Centers for Disease Control and Prevention [CDC], 2014a). There are many thousands of medications that are prescribed for numerous reasons. In addition, there are many over-the-counter (OTC) products that are also taken. Some of these medicines, such as aspirin, may be very dangerous when taken with another prescribed "blood thinning" medicine. Another example is the prescription blood thinner warfarin. Though shown to be a very effective drug, there are many thousands of ED visits related to warfarin as well. And these are just two examples. Acetaminophen toxicity also brings many thousands of people to the emergency department. All medications have risks and side effects—whether good or bad ones. I am sure you have heard some of the "direct to consumer advertising" for prescription drugs on TV. I had one patient ask me "Is this a joke?" Who would take this when the problems listed at the end of the ad are worse than the problem it was supposed to fix?" Medications have very serious benefits and very serious risks and some of these ads display this clearly!

This section seeks to make the complex issue of medications and safety more understandable from a practical perspective as you care for your caregivee/loved one. There is no question we take a lot of medications in the U.S. According to the CDC, among adults aged 60 or older "more than 76% used two or more prescription drugs and 37% used five or more" (2010).

If you remember two things as you navigate the confusing information about medications, let them be these two:

1. The pharmacist is your best resource and the expert about medications and their effects and interactions with other medications that your caregivee/loved one might be taking. It makes sense that the more drugs or medications that a person takes, the more health problems the person may have and so the more safety considerations must be assessed. Polypharmacy is a term that means the practice of administering or using multiple medications especially concurrently (as in the treatment of a single disease or of several coexisting conditions) (merriam-webster.com, n.d.). Polypharmacy has implications for everyone, as the population ages and medications are sometimes seen as the "fix" to some short- and long-term health problems. It may be true that more pills are not always better; sometimes more pills lead to more interactions. Some drugs can also cause confusion and decrease memory and may cause the patient to be misdiagnosed as having Alzheimer's disease.

2. The second thing to remember about medication safety is that it is a good idea to establish a relationship with one pharmacy and one pharmacist there who knows about ALL the medications your caregivee/loved one is

taking—from all various doctors or prescribers. Consider a certified geriatric pharmacist (http://www.ccgp.org/).

Let's look at this another way. If your caregivee/loved one is suffering from cancer, there may be several physicians and health care providers involved. For purposes of illustration, let's presume that the person has prostate cancer. The man who is sick is being followed by 1) his primary doctor or a nurse practitioner, 2) an oncologist for the cancer, 3) a radiologist for radiation treatments, 4) a surgeon for the initial prostate surgery, and 5) if he is hospitalized, perhaps a "hospitalist" who takes care of him while he is a patient in the inpatient hospital. This could be five providers writing prescriptions or otherwise recommending medications for care. This can get particularly problematic when planning for discharge and for care back at home and this may be the same time the caregiver will be assimilating the information about other care after discharge as well, such as care for a surgical site. There could be even more physicians ordering medications or treatments (such as oxygen) if one doctor is off and "covering" for another. Either way, it is very important that the caregiver be the person that knows the "correct" list of prescription medications, OTC products, herbs, lotions, and all other medications that your caregivee/loved one uses. It would be reasonable to presume that the doctors and other providers are all communicating and coordinating with each other about this man's care and his medications. Sadly, all too often, this is not true. This is where the caregiver is so important—so that there is one person who acts as their advocate or patient's representative, who is knowledgeable about the caregivee/loved one and their unique history: they have and manage the correct and up-to-date medication list, know the patient's usual personality, and honors and supports their unique needs and wishes.

The accurate medication list is very important for safety, communication, and quality reasons. This is because communication factors are thought to be a common cause of errors. Here is where your local pharmacist comes in handy—the pharmacist is an expert and has access to systems that can help identify possible medication interactions. There are a few kinds of "interactions." The most common is called "drug-drug" and this is where one drug "interacts" (and usually not in a good way) with another. There can also be "drug-food" interactions. One of the most common drug-food interactions is the grapefruit-drug interaction. There are a number of medications that may react negatively with grapefruit juice. Generally, this includes some medications used for treating cholesterol, infections, and other health problems. This has implications for many who drink grapefruit juice—so be sure and ask your pharmacist/doctor if it could be impacting your caregivee/loved one's specific drug regimen. In addition, be aware that most pharmacies have a computer system that can run all drug-drug interactions on the medications they are providing for your loved one and also list all of the key side effects for each medication.

For purposes of clarity, a "regimen," in this case a drug regimen, means the medications that your caregivee/loved one takes regularly as recommended or prescribed by a member of the health care team. There are sample forms to help keep track and up-to-date on your caregivee's/loved one's medication regimen in Chapter Five: Creating and Maintaining a Care Notebook or Binder (Or Take This with You to the

Doctor, Nurse, or Hospital!). Keep a copy of the latest medication list somewhere in the front section of that notebook or binder so it is easily accessible when needed. In addition, it is a good idea to keep it with the caregivee/loved one or in the caregiver's wallet or purse.

Medication Reconciliation—What Is It and Why Is It Important?

It is very important that you keep and maintain an accurate and up-to-date list of all medications, including OTC products and any herbs, lotions, and/or vitamins that your caregivee/loved one takes. All these products, depending on what it is and the dose and usage, may cause interactions, or negative effects. This list should also include any liquids, powders, or creams. These "topical" products (applied to the skin) are usually absorbed through the skin. Another safety tip is to speak very clearly and write clearly (legibly) when communicating about medications including "PRN" or as needed medications. This is so everyone involved in the care understands the medication to which you are referring. Simply put, medication reconciliation means the "process of identifying the most accurate list of all medications that the patient is taking, including name, dosage, frequency, and route, by comparing the medical record to an external list of medications obtained from a patient, hospital, or other provider" (Centers for Medicare and Medicaid Services [CMS], 2014). This medication reconciliation process is one fundamental way to keep track of the correct medications that can be coordinated and confirmed across care settings. There are so many "moving parts" in health care. This is one way to ensure that your caregivee/loved one has the correct medications on the list and that none are forgotten, missing, and/or should no longer be taken (such as when they have been discontinued). In this way, the accurate and correct dose and other important details and parameters are verified and confirmed—and this should occur in every health care setting, the hospital setting, the emergency department, in home care, the doctor's office—wherever care is provided!

Even in hospitals, there are "drug errors," caused by "sound-alike" and "look-alike" drugs. So try not to use abbreviations when talking about medications. This is another way in which clarity helps keep people safe—the less anyone has to guess or assume (not all abbreviations mean the same thing to everyone everywhere) the better for safety and quality. There are no dumb questions when it comes to medications! Always check the medication when you pick up a new prescription for your caregivee/loved one. Check that it is what the doctor or nurse told you they were going to "call in" to the pharmacy or what was written on the paper prescription. If there is any question, speak with the pharmacist, who can better address concerns since they have direct access to the ordering physician. Make sure you note or verbalize any allergies to the doctor who is ordering the new medication, and, if possible, do this before it is ordered.

When there is a new medication added to the regimen, ask the doctor: What is the name of the new medicine? What is the new medicine for (or what is it treating/for exactly)? Am I supposed to wake my caregivee/loved one to take this medication? (An example is the prescription bottle says 4 times a day—is that 4 times in the daytime or spread out over 24 hours and so really every 6 hours?) What is the exact way to take this medicine? How long will your caregivee/loved one be on this new medication? When should it be stopped? If a dose is forgotten, what do you do? What side effects can be expected? (For example, it may make your caregivee/loved one very tired—then you know you have to watch carefully that they do not fall.) Are there any special storage considerations, such as refrigeration? Who should you call if there is a problem? The pharmacist will know this information. The more you know and understand, the better caregiver and advocate you can be for your caregivee/loved one! It is always encouraged that you write notes down in your care notebook or binder to help you remember when the new medication was started, why, and any other pertinent information. Of course, observe the caregivee/loved one after any new medication has been started and call the doctor for any rashes, dizziness, or other problems or effects. Some people are very allergic to some medications, and even some that they have taken for years—like penicillin. If your caregivee/loved one has trouble breathing or other serious side effects—call 9-1-1 and, if possible, give the drug bottle to the responders so they also know the medication.

The Beers List for Older Adults—What Is It?

Consumers need to be educated more about health care— after all, it is your body and health, and that of your caregivee/loved one. As the population ages, the Beers Criteria has important implications as we all seek to age well and age in place in our homes if we can. The Beers List is a set of medications and pharmacologic features that generally are viewed as potentially inappropriate medications. This list was first published in 1991 and has since been updated. This list has been used to help improve the safety of medications being prescribed for and used by older adults. These are drugs that have been shown to have increased adverse effects for that age group. They might contribute to polypharmacy and where the Beers List identifies potential risks, these risks might outweigh the drug's benefits. The Beers list can be accessed at https://www.dcri.org/trial-participation/the-beers-list. If your caregivee/loved one is on one of these medications, it is important that they keep taking it until you have a conversation with the prescriber/health care professional to discuss the concern and plan.

As the body ages, the organs that process medications age as well. This can mean our bodies cannot eliminate medications as quickly leading to higher "active medications" remaining in the body. This can increase the risk of side effects. Let's look at an example. One of the medications on the Beers list is diazepam, which is the generic name for Valium. This drug is known to cause sleepiness, confusion, weakness, and sometimes more serious side effects. Now consider that a small, frail older woman is placed on this medication for "sleep." She has a history of falls, which she hides from most family members (which is not unusual). This drug's side effects could contribute to falls and may add to other health problems that are already known in this patient. When added to the medication regimen of the woman in this example, the medication chosen for sleep or anxiety (this is just an example) could cause symptoms and problems that may not improve her health and functioning.

Falls

Falls are a large and multifactorial problem, especially in the older adult population. More women than men fall. Women are also more likely to have osteoporosis and are more likely to have fractures from falling than men. The health system is moving toward a more "health-focused" model as opposed to a predominately "illness-focused" model. The future trajectory is that health care moves toward preventing untoward or preventable events, such as falls, when it can. Medications are just one part of this big picture. In this case, the prevention of just one factor for falls, medication, was used to illustrate this connection. Though not all falls can be prevented, caregivers should be aware of the risks and the caregivee/loved one should be assessed for risk. Falls are discussed later in this chapter in more detail. Proactive approaches can only help improve care for older adults and patients of all ages in the years ahead.

Other Medication Safety Considerations

When the patient is a child, it is even more important than ever that dosing and dosages be accurate. Pediatric dosages are usually calculated by weight, and other factors as well. Like adults, sick or debilitated children may be on many medications. Again, the caregiver, oftentimes the parents or a home care nurse, must be aware of the detailed management that comes with a complex medication and care regimen. Again, medication reconciliation is important. Also proper measuring devices and accurate dosing is very important. Ask the pharmacist about droppers, spoons, and exactly how much to give. In addition, there may be other children in the household and so the medications need to be stored safely.

If there are children and/or grandchildren who come to visit your caregivee/loved one—know that the pharmacy can put the medications in childproof bottles. Still, place the bottles in a safe place where children cannot easily reach or access them. Just because the cap says it is childproof does not always mean that it is! In addition, when you clean out old medications, whether prescription or over-the-counter, it is very important that they NOT be flushed down the toilet. Sadly, many fish and other species that live in the ocean have been found to contain antidepressants and other human drugs in their blood. For more information, visit www.epa.gov/ppcp/ or call the Safe Drinking Water Hotline at (800) 426-4791. The FDA also provides information about disposing of medications: http://www.fda.gov/ForConsumers/ConsumerUpdates/ucm101653.htm. Some communities also hold events where outdated or no longer in use medications can be properly disposed of.

Think about safety and how to avoid a problem wherever possible!

E—Environment of Care

The home is a very unique setting for health care. If we think about it, it is where health decisions, like lifestyle choices, are made every day. This includes things like what to eat for breakfast, lunch, and dinner; what snacks to have; how much salt to add to food; and/or how often to take a walk. Lots of these seemingly small daily decisions add up to weeks, months, and then years and help lead us toward good health or not so good health. The above discussion about medications included a section about certain types of medications that may be potentially inappropriate in older adults and the Beers List. Sadly, certain medications can contribute to falls. As stated above, falls are a complex phenomenon and so whatever the reason, it is prudent to always try to avoid them, whenever possible. It is well known that falls are the leading cause of injuries for those over age 65 (CDC, 2014b). One report stated that it is estimated that an older adult is seen in an emergency department every 14 seconds for a fall-related problem/injury (National Council on Aging [NCOA], n.d.).

Falls—Complexity in Action

- According to the National Institute on Aging, six out of every 10 falls happen at home (NIH Senior Health, n.d.). The following are some tips adapted from Go4Life (See in resources listed at the end of this chapter; http://go4life.nia .nih.gov/).
- Remove anything that could cause someone to trip or slip while walking, such as throw rugs in living areas or kitchens, bath mats in bathrooms, etc.
- Clutter, small furniture, pet bowls, electrical or phone cords, and throw rugs can cause falls.
- Arrange furniture so that there is plenty of room to walk freely with assistive device, wheelchair, cane, etc. Remove items from stairs and hallways. Consider a gate at the top of stairs.
- Use caution with small pets that can get under foot.
- Sit in chairs/couches where feet can touch the floor. Hips should be equal to or above your knees. Consider using furniture lifts if the surface is too low.

- Avoid wet floors and clean up spills right away. Use non-slip items in the bathroom.
- Put non-slip strips or a rubber mat on the floor of the bathtub or shower.
- Do not walk in socks, stockings or non-rubber soled slippers!
- Make sure there is enough lighting in each room, on stairs, at entrances, and on outdoor walkways.
- Place a lamp next to the bed along with nightlights in the bathroom, hallways, and kitchen.
- Keep a flashlight by the bed in case the power goes out and you need to get up at night.
- Encourage your caregivee/loved one to wear their glasses and hearing aids.
- Stay as physically active as possible. Lower body strength and balance exercises can help prevent falls.
- Consider having your caregivee/loved one attend balance and strengthening exercise classes at a local senior center—these classes are sometimes taught sitting down and the instructor is sometimes a nurse or a physical therapist.
- Walking and stretching exercises are also important to help prevent falls.
- Use a cane or walker or other equipment to help with balance if needed. A cane can improve balance, and canes have gotten much more fashionable. A nurse friend decorated hers to match her daughter's wedding party—she won the cane award by gluing eyelet lace and painting the cane purple!
- Consider a personal emergency response system or some type of emergency call.
- Be very careful when it is winter and there is ice and

snow—consider only going out with a trusted friend for support and, even then, be very careful!

Driving: A Difficult Topic—
When to Give Up the Keys

A discussion about safety would not be complete without the topic of driving. It can be a very hard topic to broach with your caregivee/loved one. But, as the caregiver, you will know when it is time. The following are just a few changes that may identify a change in function, ability, or capability that may indicate it is time to stop driving. This is not an all-inclusive list.

Some indicators include:

- The person has been diagnosed with dementia or Alzheimer's and has memory loss. This may occur when familiar places become difficult to locate.
- When you have driven with them and feel unsafe, perhaps they drive too fast or slow or cuss at other drivers. Or you may notice that others will no longer drive with them.
- If vision and depth perception becomes a problem— sometimes this may be verbalized as the "signs are too small" and "too far away."
- Perhaps they are on a medication where the bottle has a notation "not to drive or work with heavy machinery." Ask your pharmacist if any of the medications your caregivee/ loved one is on precludes driving. This information may help with the decision and the discussion.
- More information is better as it helps provide a realistic picture of the driver's capability and ability.

Here is one example. Mr. Smith is 89 years old and on numerous medications for various ailments and health problems. He was asked by his daughter to meet her at the local grocery store. The daughter was noticing that he seemed more forgetful in the past few weeks. When her father did not show up at the designated time at the grocery store, she found him still at home. He had forgotten their conversation in the time between her call that morning and the 15 minutes later when he was to leave to meet her. Such a situation raised significant safety concerns. And this was not the first time he had forgotten to meet her somewhere. The father was seen by his doctor and it was decided that he should no longer drive. In fact, the daughter was surprised that her father verbalized relief at this decision and stated, "I have been worried that I might hurt someone; everyone drives too fast." Adult children or others must then become the drivers and errand runners on top of other roles and responsibilities. There is no easy solution to this problem. Each family must work out how to take Dad out to get groceries, get a haircut, play cards at the senior center, and other activities. Whatever the solution, it is important that the caregivee/loved one not be isolated and stuck in their home from a socialization and a quality of life perspective. The older adult may need to feel that you want to do this and that they are not a burden.

One useful resource is at the National Institute of Health's Senior Health site. There is a very useful section entitled "Older Drivers" that lists how aging affects driving and reviews why and how driving is "A Complex Task" (n.d.). It also lists "Common Mistakes" of older drivers including: "failing to yield the right of way, failing to stay in lane, misjudging the time or distance needed to turn in front of traffic, failing to stop completely at a stop sign, and speeding or driving too slowly." They also report that the risk of "crashes rises with age, especially after age 75. Studies show that older drivers are more likely to be involved in certain types of crashes" than others. The more likely are: "at intersections (usually in the vehicle that is struck), in which the front of one vehicle hits the side of the other vehicle, and where the older driver is merging and the other vehicle is traveling faster or is in the driver's blind spot."

Types of Healthcare Provided at Home

Your caregivee/loved one might need care in the home, depending on their unique healthcare needs. There are many people who are cared for at home. Kinds of care provided in the home care setting are home care and hospice, as well as other services. Some of these services might be paid for by insurance and other services might be what is called "private pay" or "private duty." Private care, for an example, would be when the caregiver/family employs an aide or a companion to be with your caregivee/loved one while you work during the day. This would be a service that you choose and pay for privately.

Insurance coverage for care at home is variable and, generally, sparse. Sadly, Medicare pays for a very limited amount of "skilled" care in the home. There are certain criteria that the older adult must meet to "qualify" for home care services. This includes that they need a "skilled" level of care, that the skilled care meets the coverage, and other criteria for payment; that there is physician certification, clear evidence that the patient is "homebound," and that leaving the home is a considerable and taxing effort and of short duration.

Homebound does not mean that they no longer want to drive or do not want to go out for other reasons. It means that because of a medical reason the person cannot generally leave their home. Examples include a patient who is bedbound and at end of life or a patient who is primarily confined (due to medical reasons) to the home from diabetes who requires a prosthesis and needs a nurse and/or a physical therapist may qualify.

Qualifying for home care is based on the individualized findings of the data collected from a very comprehensive assessment performed in the patient's home. The admitting home health agency (HHA) nurse and physician evaluate for the "need." It is important to note that Medicare is a medical insurance program and like any insurance program there are coverage (and other) criteria. "Medical necessity" means that the care is just that—based on medical need as defined by Medicare coverage and its rules and regulations, not care for social or convenience reasons.

Some questions to ask before you and your caregivee/loved one leave the hospital or doctor's office include:

- What amount of care will be needed once home?
- Was a referral to a home health or hospice agency made? Does your doctor or other care provider think you qualify for these services? If a referral was made for home care, ask for the name of the home care organization and their phone number—this will be important should you need to call them and/or if no one contacts you once home and needing care.
- Will your caregivee/loved one be "homebound" once home?
- How will pain or other symptoms be controlled?

- When will your caregivee/loved one next be seen by the doctor?

If you hire an aide privately, reference and background checks are a must for safety. Questions such as: What is your background? What training do you have? What ongoing education do you participate in? These are all important. This is a complex area because some aides are employed by agencies while others are not. If your doctor makes a referral for your caregivee/loved one to a licensed or Medicare-certified home health agency there are generally rules, called the "Medicare Conditions of Participation," that must be met to receive government reimbursement (such as Medicare or Medicaid). Some states have licensure and some home health agencies are also "accredited" similar to how hospitals are accredited. These home visits are "intermittent" care. For example, a licensed visiting nurse, such as registered nurse, may come to the home for specific nursing care. This might include medication management for a short while and assuming the patient remains homebound, caring for/changing an indwelling urinary catheter, and other "skilled" services. The details are complex and the organizations usually know and explain the "rules" to patients and caregivers. Also check with your local area agency on aging for possible assistance in your area (www.n4a.org) or Eldercare Locator (http://www.eldercare .gov).

Your state government may also have another home care program covered by Medicaid. Medicaid is a health payer and a state program for those who meet state-specific criteria. Medicaid historically was "means tested," meaning one must meet certain financial criteria and rules and specific state's requirements to obtain the benefit. There are different names for Medicaid in some states, such as Medi-Cal in California, TennCare in Tennessee, and Mass Health in Massachusetts. Some of these states have special programs, such as those for very sick children. Services covered by Medicaid might include a visiting nurse; therapists, such as physical, occupational, and/or speech-language pathologists; and/or home health aides.

Hospice care is another special program and is directed to patients who are facing a life-threatening or life-limiting illness and their families/friends. That is one of the most special things about hospice care. It is not directed solely toward the patient, but also helps care for and support the caregiver—which is very important.

Like home care, hospice has specific qualifying criteria, including criteria related to prognosis. The hospice team might include the hospice nurse, the hospice physician, the patient's primary care doctor/provider, the social worker, hospice volunteers (these are volunteers who are specially trained to work with hospice patients and families), therapists, home health aides, and a chaplain or spiritual counselor. Hospices work through an interdisciplinary care team (IDT) model and are usually experts at pain and other end-of-life symptom management. In hospice, the patient's family and/or caregivers are also supported after the patient has died—through bereavement services, which help the family process their grief and loss. Hospice is also unique in that it seeks to make every day the best it can be—which is how we all should live. Some hospice patients have said that they have been given a gift because they know "about how long" they have to live and the rest of us don't, and this allows quality time with family and friends. It does make one think about how we live each and every day.

If you do have visiting nurses, hospice nurses, or other team members visit, remember that they are there to provide certain services and skills. Your specific home and environment of care can add to their effectiveness if you do the following:

- Put all pets away for the duration of the visit. Though this is a home, there are certain infection control and other aspects of care where a pet is not appropriate.
- Have the caregivee/loved one's log/notebook available.
- Turn off the TV or radio so the nurse, therapist, or other team member can hear your answers and can generally better and more clearly communicate. The nurse performs a physical assessment and so may need to carefully hear a blood pressure or heart or lung sounds.
- The nurse, aide, or therapist may carry a laptop/tablet as they must document findings—like at the hospital or the doctor's office. Facilitate this process by having a clean/ quiet area for this to be accomplished.
- Have a liquid hand soap and clean paper towels available for team members to use—they need to and will wash their hands, like at any other health care setting.
- Have all the caregivee's/loved one's medications in one place for the nurse or therapist or pharmacist to review—this is also for medication reconciliation purposes that were discussed earlier in this chapter. Have a current list of all doctors, their office addresses, and their phone numbers.
- The home care organization or hospice will have a special written "plan of care" for your caregivee/loved one. Try to keep this and all the papers that you might have signed or

been sent in one folder so that the agency nurse or therapist or aide can find that information. The aide would usually have what is called a "Home Health Aide Plan of Care" that the registered nurse completes based on the findings and the patient care needs identified. Should there be a question or concern about the care being provided, contact the organization's nursing director.

Other health-related services that might be provided at home sometimes include technology. There may be telehealth where the caregiver and patient report data (such as blood pressures, etc.) through an automated mechanism or it may be a nurse from the hospital, insurance program, or home health agency who calls and using specialized technology is able to check on the patient and caregiver. Such detailed, personalized care are efforts to improve safety and quality. There might also be a "PERS" or a Personal Emergency Response System that can alert services should there be a fall or other bad event and the person "cannot get up" or otherwise needs assistance. The use of technology in the home will only increase as home becomes the preferred setting for care.

Safety and Emergency Management Considerations

Caregivees/loved ones do best with consistency in caregivers and knowing what the days "hold in store." Unfortunately, disasters can come in many forms and disrupt our day-to-day activities and care. Because of the responsibilities that come with caregiving related to safety, it is important to talk about "emergency preparedness." Whether the heat goes out (and for more than a short time), a hurricane approaches and the family must leave, or any number of other natural or man-made disasters strike, thoughtful consideration must be given to the question "what if?" Simply put, this means there needs to be a plan. When an emergency happens, resources can be quickly strained. For many reasons, it is important to be self-sufficient and proactive. Electricity, water, telephone, and other services may be unavailable. Grocery stores may shut down as workers leave to care for their own families and make their own preparations. The Ready program has resources to help you plan (http://www.ready.gov/). Such areas as "Make A Plan," "Build A Kit," and information about knowing your risks, depending on where you live, can all be helpful. The Federal Emergency Management Agency (FEMA) also offers resources and information, plus they have an app that can be downloaded (www.fema.gov).

These considerations are even more crucial if your caregivee/loved one is bedridden or is very debilitated and must have electricity for life-sustaining technology, such as oxygen or a respirator. For example, is there a back-up generator? Carefully consider where you would go—is there a hospital or somewhere else where pre-planned arrangements can be made for transportation to sites for further care? Sometimes "sheltering in place" is not an option. If your caregivee/loved one uses electricity for life-sustaining technology, such as a ventilator, and/or is oxygen dependent, the local emergency services should be notified. Hopefully, they are already aware of the unique health needs of your caregivee/loved one—before any such emergency situation should occur. It is also prudent to have a complete set of back-up supplies, including medications, on hand and in the home should you need them. In addition to the health care specific items needed for your unique caregivee/loved ones, consider the necessary household supply kit. You and your caregivee/loved one might need to depend upon it.

Summary

Home is where most people report that they wish to be and where they wish to receive healthcare when possible. It is very different from the hospital. No one tells you what time visitors can come and go, what food is to be served and what times, that pets are not allowed, the age of visitors allowed, or what to wear. Your home is where you set the rules—it is your castle! And health care providers coming into the home must respect that basic tenet. Factors impacting safety in the home setting are numerous and as unique as the home and the people/family and pets living there. This overview presents some information and resources for the caregiver to help make it a safe(r) place for themselves and their caregivee/loved one. Like any care setting, infection control is important. The next chapter (Chapter Seven: Infection Control and Prevention Considerations) addresses some of the fundamentals of infection control in the home and across other health care settings you might encounter.

Resources for You

- The U.S. Fire Administration offers many pamphlets on their website in both English and Spanish: http://www.usfa .fema.gov/prevention/outreach/older_adults.html
- The Mayo Clinic offers a fact sheet called "Medication errors: Cut your risk with these tips": http://www

.mayoclinic.org/healthy-living/consumer-health/in-depth/
medication-errors/art-20048035

- Go4Life from the National Institute on Aging at NIH
  offers help to begin getting physically active and improving
  your diet: http://go4life.nia.nih.gov/
- The Administration for Community Living offers a resource titled "Healthy Living Tips: How Do You Know
  When It's Time to Give Up the Keys": http://www.acl.gov/
  NewsRoom/Publications/docs/HealthyLivingTips_Give
  UptheKeys.pdf
- The Centers for Disease Control and Prevention (CDC)
  in "Older Adult Drivers: Get the Facts" lists a lot of great
  information, including that "age-related declines in vision
  and cognitive functioning (ability to reason and remember),
  as well as physical changes, may affect some older adults'
  driving abilities": http://www.cdc.gov/motorvehiclesafety/
  older_adult_drivers/adult-drivers_factsheet.html
- The Centers for Disease Control and Prevention (CDC)
  also offers a site called "Healthy Homes" to help support making homes healthy and safe through checking
  things like water and air quality: http://www.cdc.gov/
  healthyhomes/
- The CDC also has a page on "Adults and Older Adult Adverse Drug Events": http://www.cdc.gov/MedicationSafety/
  Adult_AdverseDrugEvents.html
- For further information about medication safety, visit
  the Centers for Disease Control and Prevention's "Medication Safety Program" website at http://www.cdc.gov/
  medicationsafety/
- The National Institute on Aging (NIA) offers a resource
  called "Older Drivers" which includes a practical discussion

about older drivers that reviews fundamental changes in the body, vision, reactions, health, medications: www.nia.nih .gov/print/health/publication/older-drivers

- *The Checklist Manifesto: How to Get Things Right* by Atul Gawande is a book about how checklists can help us in every day as well as professional life.
- Atul Gawande also wrote a book called *Being Mortal*, published in 2014, about how medicine has an important role to play not just in prolonging life, but also in helping it end well.
- In addition, Atul Gawande has an article in *The New Yorker* called "Overkill: An avalanche of unnecessary medical care is harming patients physically and financially. What can we do about it?":http://www.newyorker.com/ magazine/2015/05/11/overkill-atul-gawande
- The National Center on Elder Abuse from the Administration on Aging offers resources about elder abuse: http:// www.ncea.aoa.gov/
- The Agency for Healthcare Research and Quality (AHRQ) offers a guide called "20 Tips to Help Prevent Medical Errors": http://www.ahrq.gov/patients-consumers/care-planning/errors/20tips/index.html
- Consumer Health Choices, from Consumer Reports Health, offers a guide called "Hospital Hazards Four practices that can harm older people": http://consumer healthchoices.org/wp-content/uploads/2015/06/Choosing WiselyHospitalRoundupAAN-ER.pdf
- Medicare.gov offers a "Guide to Choosing a Hospital": http://www.medicare.gov/Publications/Pubs/pdf/10181.pdf
- The U.S. Food and Drug Administration (FDA) has a guide available to help "Avoid Food-Drug Interactions":

http://www.fda.gov/downloads/Drugs/ResourcesForYou/
Consumers/BuyingUsingMedicineSafely/EnsuringSafe
UseofMedicine/GeneralUseofMedicine/UCM229033.pdf
- The Complex Child E-Magazine offers information about
  caregiving for children: http://www.complexchild.com/
- The U.S. Food and Drug Administration (FDA) offers a
  list of "Four Medication Safety Tips for Older Adults":
  http://www.fda.gov/ForConsumers/ConsumerUpdates/
  ucm399834.htm

References

AARP. (2010). Aging in Place. Retrieved from http://www.aarp.org/
home-garden/livable-communities/info-07-2010/aging-in-place.html

Centers for Disease Control and Prevention (CDC). (2014a). Medication
Safety Program. Retrieved from http://www.cdc.gov/MedicationSafety/
program_focus_activities.html

Centers for Disease Control and Prevention (CDC). (2014b). Falls Among
Older Adults: An Overview. Retrieved from http://www.cdc.gov/
homeandrecreationalsafety/falls/adultfalls.html

Centers for Disease Control and Prevention (CDC). (2010). Prescription
Drug Use Continues to Increase: U.S. Prescription Drug Data for
2007-2008. Retrieved from http://www.cdc.gov/nchs/data/databriefs/
db42.htm

Centers for Medicare and Medicaid Services (CMS). (2014). Eligible
Professional Meaningful Use Menu Set Measures Measure 6 of 9.
Retrieved from http://www.cms.gov/Regulations-and-Guidance/
Legislation/EHRIncentivePrograms/downloads/7_Medication_
Reconciliation.pdf

Garrouste-Orgeas, M, Philippart, F, Bruel, C, Max, A, Lau, N, Misset, B.
(2012). Overview of medical errors and adverse events. *Annals of Intensive Care*, 2:2.

merriam-webster.com. (n.d.). polypharmacy. Retrieved from http://www
.merriam-webster.com/dictionary/polypharmacy

National Council on Aging (NCOA). (n.d.). Falls Prevention: Fact Sheet.

Retrieved from http://www.ncoa.org/press-room/fact-sheets/falls-prevention-fact-sheet.html

National Fire Protection Association. (2008). Fires and Burns Involving Home Medical Oxygen. Retrieved from file:///C:/Users/Britosaurus/Downloads/OSOxygen.pdf

National Institute on Aging (NIA). (n.d.) Older Drivers. Retrieved from http://www.nia.nih.gov/print/health/publication/older-drivers

NIH Senior Health. (n.d.) Falls and Older Adults. Retrieved from http://nihseniorhealth.gov/falls/homesafety/01.html

U.S. Fire Administration. (2012). Fire Safety Checklist. Retrieved from http://www.usfa.fema.gov/downloads/pdf/publications/fa-221.pdf

Infection Control and
Prevention Considerations

Hospital patients acquire an estimated 722,000 infections each year (Centers for Disease Control and Prevention [CDC], 2014a). That is about one infection for every 25 patients (CDC, 2014a). Infections in the hospital and in the community have been featured in newspapers and on TV. There have been stories about "scopes" used internally that were not cleaned properly and as a result infections were transmitted. There have been stories about Ebola, about MRSA (methicillin-resistant *Staphylococcus aureus*), and "superbugs." Superbugs are multi-drug-resistant bacteria. There is no question that these stories are scary because anything that threatens our health and lives is scary. However, we should also increase efforts to further prevent the acquiring and transmission of infection to others. Caregivers have an important role related to infection prevention and control (IPC). This chapter presents a broad overview of some of the fundamentals of effective infection control and prevention.

According to the Centers for Disease Control and Prevention (CDC), antibiotics and similar drugs, called antimicrobial agents, have been in use for the last 70 years. Antibiotics are prescribed when a person has an infection, such as a bacterial urinary tract infection or pneumonia. Sadly, many times, antibiotics have been prescribed for a "virus" such as the cold, where it will not be effective because antibiotics do not treat viruses. Because antibiotics have now been used for so long and so widely, the infectious organisms that the antibiotics were designed to kill have instead adapted to them, which makes the drugs less effective and the bacteria stronger. "Each year at least 2 million people become infected with bacteria that are resistant to antibiotics also called anti-microbial resistance, and at least 23,000 people die each year as a direct result of these infections" (CDC, 2014b). What this means practically, for us as healthcare consumers, is that some antibiotics may not work and that antibiotics should only be prescribed when someone has a bacterial infection.

Infections are diseases that are caused by bacteria or viruses that are microscopic, meaning they cannot be seen by the human eye. Infections are spread when the organism, such as bacteria or viruses, are "carried" from one site or person to another. One example is when we touch a doorknob and touch our eyes—in this example, the organisms can get on the hands and then be passed to ourselves by touching our eyes. Next in the chain, a colleague or friend is seen and we "shake" hands. Then, we pass the organisms on to others who we touch with our hands. Hopefully, they wash their hands and stop this "chain of transmission!" In fact, think about moving away from shaking hands, especially in health care settings. This is why sometimes you will see doctors and/ or nurses in the work setting with their hands behind their backs or crossed in front of their chest. They are working to protect you and your caregivee/loved one! Join the initiative to stop shaking hands in healthcare settings.

Hand washing or "hand hygiene" is the single most im-portant way we can protect our caregivee/loved one from catching a cold or the flu (influenza) or other infection. The organisms in our environment can be spread in different ways and do not always make us sick. This "getting sick" depends on many factors. Regardless, do not touch your eyes, nose, or mouth without first washing your hands. Be vigilant to protect yourself and your caregivee/loved one as they already have health problems and may not "bounce back" from some infections. They may already have a compromised immune system, which means they may not have the ability to "fight off" infections like healthy people. Many germs can live for hours/days on surfaces like tables, doorknobs, or equipment.

The phrase "standard precautions" describes the methods used in health care settings designed to help protect patients and staff from all these microscopic germs and organisms. Many infections are spread before it is known that they are present, or before people exhibit symptoms that they are even sick. It is for this reason that all health care workers must use these standard precautions to protect themselves and patients, to decrease the spread of infections. These standard precautions are guidelines that are used whenever you and your caregivee/loved one go into any health care setting, including the emergency department, an outpatient clinic, the hospital, and others.

Handwashing: The Basics

According to the CDC, handwashing is one of the most important things you can do to prevent infection (2014c). "Hand washing is one of the most effective and most overlooked ways to stop disease. Soap and water work well to kill germs. Wash for at least 20 seconds and rub your hands briskly. Disposable hand wipes or gel sanitizers also work well" (MedlinePlus, n.d.). Handwashing should always occur: before and after providing any care to your caregivee/loved one, before and after any meal preparations, after using the restroom or toilet, after coughing or sneezing or blowing your nose, anytime the hands are visibly soiled, and other times as needed. This also includes before and after eating and drinking—such as going to the hospital cafeteria, or other areas in the hospital setting. When using gloves for care, remove the gloves and immediately wash your hands! When in doubt, wash your hands! This recommendation does not end when the patient is at a health care facility—in fact, it may be more important! There are "bugs" and infections seen in hospitals and other care settings that are very dangerous. For this reason, watch that the health care provider, such as a nurse or a doctor or anyone else providing direct patient care, wash their hands before they touch or care for you or your caregivee/loved one. If you don't see them wash their hands, ask them! You may have noticed that there are sinks and soap and paper towels in most exam rooms, whether the emergency department, a doctor's office, or a hospital room. There are also usually hand sanitizer dispensers available for health care providers and visitors in various departments and at entry ways. All of these opportunities to wash one's hands remind us about the importance of hand hygiene.

The topic of infections and their prevention in hospitals is a very big area of concern and is oftentimes a focus for quality improvement. Quality improvement means simply that the organization is trying to improve quality of care and operations. This is usually done through vigilant assessment and identification of patients and infections, in-depth analysis of the problem, and then efforts initiated toward future prevention. And then that cycle continues toward further performance improvements, such as a reduction in infections. Infections can take many forms and be very serious, sometimes resulting in death.

Health care providers should practice regular hand hygiene at key points in time to disrupt the transmission of microorganisms to patients including: before patient contact (this is why it is important that you watch for this); after contact with blood, body fluids, or contaminated surfaces (even if gloves are worn); before and after invasive procedures; and after removing gloves (wearing gloves is not enough to prevent the transmission of pathogens in healthcare settings) (CDC, 2014a).

You must be proactive and speak up if you do not see your caregivee/loved one's doctor or nurse wash their hands! They should also apply gloves if they will be closely examining any kind of open wound or open skin area. The nurses and doctors and others are usually very busy—but speak up and say, "I am sorry, I did not see you wash your hands." You might add that your caregivee/loved one is frail and just getting over a cold or whatever; you just need to see them wash their hands.

Consider carrying hand wipes or alcohol-based gel with you and clean your hands and your caregiver/loved one's while there. Think of all the things that one touches at a doctor's office—the exam table, doorknobs, the weight scale, the counter at check-in and checkout, and more! The more proactive you can be by valuing IPC and hand hygiene, the better. If the doctor or nurse gets upset or otherwise shows displeasure, that is okay. You may be helping them in their efforts for quality improvement related to IPC!

Coughing and Germs

Always carry clean tissues in your purse or in your "to go" bag or backpack or whatever you carry to the doctor's office or any other health care setting. Cover your nose and mouth with a tissue when you cough or sneeze. Do not sneeze or cough into your hands. Cover your sneeze or cough with your sleeve or your elbow. Throw the tissue into the trash. Wash your hands immediately and try not to touch anything. Besides hand gel, consider carrying those "wet wipes" for use when you cannot get to a sink. And then—when you can get to a sink—use soap and water, and wash your hands!

Efforts about IPC are even more important in winter time when the flu (influenza) is present. Actions include getting vaccinated for the flu, staying away from sick or infected people, staying home from work and not spreading your germs, eating right, and getting plenty of sleep and exercise. While contagious bugs and viruses are active and around all year, fall and winter are when many people are most vulnerable because people spend more time indoors. Flu viruses spread mainly by droplets sprayed or dispersed when people with the flu cough, sneeze, or talk. The flu virus can also live on hard surfaces like doorknobs, menus, and others (CDC, 2013). A person might also get the flu by touching a surface or object that has the flu virus on it. In the 2013–2014 season, there were 35.4 million influenza-associated illnesses, 14.6 medically attended (saw the doctor about) flu illnesses, and 314,000 hospitalizations due to flu (CDC, 2014d).

Organisms Can Be Spread in Five Ways

1. Airborne—This means passed from one place or person to another through the air (airborne or droplet), such as by sneezing or coughing. Examples of airborne diseases are measles, the flu, a cold, and tuberculosis.

2. Sexual—This means passed through sexual contact like "wet" kissing (kissing with an exchange of body fluids), sexual intercourse, or other sexual behaviors. Examples include herpes, hepatitis B and C, HIV, syphilis, and chlamydia.

3. Oral—This means passed from one person to another by the sharing of food or drinks or eating utensils. Mononucleosis as an example of this type of infection.

4. Food Handling—This is the most common way to spread infection when proper hand washing or hygiene is not used. An example of an infection passed by improper handling is *Escherichia coli* (an organism present in fecal matter, bowel movements, feces, poorly stored food [which has either been stored at the wrong temperature or been contaminated by another substance]).

5. Sharing—This includes using razors, drinks, ointments, and toothbrushes that belong to someone else or that someone else has used. An example of something commonly spread this way is some kinds of Hepatitis.

However they are spread, knowing how they are transmitted can be the key to staying healthy. IPC is key to stopping the transmission of germs, bacteria, and viruses. The above are only some examples of diseases spread by germs, bacteria, and viruses. There are some infections that are usually only seen in hospitals or other healthcare settings. Your doctor is the expert on any infections, the antibiotics needed, and the plan for care and recovery. When in doubt, or if there are questions, always ask the doctor any questions you have about your caregivee/loved one and IPC. Most hospitals also have "infection preventionists"—this may be a specially trained nurse or doctor who is an expert about IPC.

When Your Caregivee/Loved One Goes to the Hospital

There are times when a hospitalization cannot be avoided. When this happens, it is very important that the caregiver be observant and be a good "visitor" while there. This includes: observing that hand hygiene is done before any care or inter-action with your caregivee/loved one or reminding/asking the health care team member who does not do this if they have washed their hands?

If there are other family members or visitors coming in—ask that they wash their hands frequently too. Consider purchasing some small alcohol handwashing products for just this purpose and give them as "gifts." This could be the best gift your caregivee/loved one gets! If someone thinks you are weird or overzealous, try and explain that the patient may not have a strong immune system—and consider referring them to some of the CDC resources at the end of this chapter for further reading about the importance of good hygiene in all settings.

Be particularly aware and alert about infections and their transmission if your caregivee/loved one has a wound (either from surgery or a pressure ulcer [what used to be called a bedsore]), an indwelling urinary catheter, a "venous catheter," which is a catheter in the vein or intravenous "IV," or any other wound or open site in the skin. All of these are areas that can become infected.

Be vigilant in observation, reporting any changes you see or changes reported to you by your caregivee/loved one. Communication to and with the staff is key. It is okay to be seen as a "squeaky wheel." Advocate for your caregivee/loved one. Just be pleasant (bring chocolates or donuts?) and usually the health care team members will understand that you are doing your best to protect your patient from Healthcare-associated infections (HAIs). They also have this same goal and your speaking up helps them in this quest!

Hospital patients often have "tubes placed in their veins to deliver medications or take blood samples" (healthfinder.gov, 2014). One recent study suggests that doctors do not always know about their patients having one or more of these tubes. This study of doctors at three large U.S. hospitals "found that 21% were unaware that a patient under their care had a central venous catheter—a tube placed in a large vein in the neck, chest, arm or groin" (healthfinder.gov, 2014).

The longer catheters stay in, the greater the risk of developing problems. Make sure to communicate to the doctors and nurses if your caregivee/loved one has any kind of catheter, tube, IV, or access "port" in place. This might include a central line, a gastrostomy tube, a urinary or suprapubic catheter—any tube that your caregivee/loved one has in/on their body, even if not being actively "used" at the time. Ask them when it can be removed. If the site has been getting on-going dressing changes or other care, perhaps from a visiting nurse or the hospice nurse, tell the hospital team when the dressing was last changed and the usual process for changing. Each dressing should be dated! Be proactive and ask the care team to date any dressings they change.

As discussed in Chapter Four: Advocacy: Your Role in Communication and Coordination, it is encouraged to repeat important information to help ensure that all team members are communicating and knowledgeable about your patient's unique needs. This is important because another doctor, perhaps a specialist or a doctor from the skilled nursing facility, may have ordered this tube and the hospital doctors do not know about it. Whenever you are in another care setting, such as the emergency department, tell the doctor and nurse if your caregivee/loved one has a port or other access site, or any kind of tube or catheter or any potentially communicable illness so the care team knows and a problem can be avoided.

If your caregivee/loved one has a catheter, whether for drawing blood or for urinary drainage reasons, ask when the catheter(s) can be removed. Of course, some patients may need catheters long-term; it all depends on the patient and their unique health care situation, needs, and problems. One example could be that a patient is at end of life and the urinary catheter is a needed comfort measure. Also, if blood is taken from the catheter or a urine sample from the urinary catheter, watch that the sample or specimen is labeled while you are there. This can help prevent a "mix-up" and helps ensure that the specimen is your caregivee/loved one's. This is just another quality "check" that you, as patient advocate, can participate in.

If a nurse or doctor comes in to give a medication, such as an antibiotic—particularly by infusion or injection—ask what the medication is, what it is for or treating, and who it is for. This may sound fundamental, but because hospitals are such busy places and the patient turnover can be high, this all adds to the complexity of care because there are lots of "moving parts." The point is, make sure that it is the right medication for your caregivee/loved one.

If your caregivee/loved one has surgery, watch for the following:

1. If they may have special stockings or technology that "pumps" their legs, that they are encouraged and helped to be "up" or "out of bed" or "dangled" at the side of the bed. These measures are to help prevent blood clots and help muscles and other systems stay strong and healthy.

2. That they are encouraged to cough and deep breathe regularly; this is to help prevent pneumonia.

3. That they are encouraged to drink water (if allowed) and urinate, which is to help prevent a urinary tract infection (UTI).

4. Watch that the surgical wound is being assessed/observed and, as caregiver, watch for any signs of infection, such as redness, fever, odor, a saturated dressing, a missed dressing change, or other signs as instructed by the care team. Ask the nurses, doctors, or surgeon what you can do to help!

Comfort is also an important part of post-surgical care, so ask for pain medications and/or anti-vomiting medications (called antiemetics) when needed. Remember that when people take pain medications, they may become very constipated. Ask the doctor or nurse if your caregivee/loved one is on medications or a regimen that may cause constipation, and the plan to prevent and treat it.

Also, for safety, be sure to watch your caregivee/loved one when they get up into a chair at the bedside. Escort them as needed based on their care needs. Falls can be a problem in hospitals and other settings and prevention is key. This may be particularly true for older adults who may become disoriented and confused when away from home. The medications, bright lights in the hospital room, noises/sounds in the hospitals, and many other factors may contribute to falls.

Your goal must be clear and focused—to get your caregivee/loved one out of the hospital as soon and as safely as you can. Once back at home, continue your good hand hygiene and other infection control habits.

Similarly, like hospitals, nursing homes and assisted living facilities also have serious infections reported. Over three million Americans reside in nursing homes and nearly one million reside in assisted living facilities. According to the CDC, "1 to 3 million serious infections occur every year in these facilities. Infections include urinary tract infection, diarrheal diseases, antibiotic-resistant staph infections and many others. Infections are a major cause of hospitalization and death; as many as 380,000 people die of the infections in LTCFs every year" (CDC, 2015). LTCF stands for long-term care facility.

Being a Good Visitor

- Hospitals, nursing homes, and other care settings may be short-staffed. And let's be honest—it is the nurses who care for patients 24 hours a day, 7 days a week. This being short-staffed may impact the care of your caregivee/loved one. Be nice to the nurses! (Bring candy or donuts!)

- Do not sit on the patient's bed or touch/handle the medical equipment unless you have been instructed to do so by a staff member. Sometimes there is education provided in the hospital to help you with the transition back to home.
- Use the public bathrooms in the facility. The bathrooms are for the patient and/or the roommate only.
- If you notice dust or dirt in the room, speak with the nursing supervisor.
- There may be a roommate, so be very respectful. Use a soft, quiet tone of voice when speaking. Leave the area to talk on a cellphone. (Cellphones may be not allowed in certain areas.) People are very sick in hospitals and may be at the end-of-life—they and their family and friends need quiet times and spaces.
- Most importantly, do not visit the hospital if you are sick or recently "getting over" something! People in hospitals are very sick and they may not have an immune system strong enough to fight a "bug." You would not want someone exposing you or your caregivee/loved one to an infection so do the same—make it okay to stay home and keep your germs to yourself!
- Personal protective equipment (PPE) will be used by hospital team members. This may include gloves for any hands-on patient contact, goggles, face masks, aprons, gowns, foot coverings, or others. You may be asked to "gown and glove up" in some cases. It all depends, based on the patient and their unique health problems. Read any signage posted near the door BEFORE entering. You may have to see the nurse at the nursing station for any questions or specific instructions.

- Patients are very sick. Unless you are the caregiver, limit your visits. Patients are in the hospital to rest and get better.
- Once back home, your caregivee/love one may be visited by a home care or a hospice nurse. These nurses will also practice IPC, such as hand hygiene. Identify a clean sink area for the nurse supplied with liquid hand soap and paper towels. Also have trash bags for the disposal of dirty items such as dressings. For IPC reasons, any pets should be kept out of the patient care area during care and the nurse visit. The nurses will also be using PPE such as gloves. Again, if they do not, speak up!
- Do not hesitate to point out the handwashing stations to family and friends. A simple "You can wash your hands here" can convey the message in a way that is not offensive.
- Standard precautions are effective and important tools to prevent and control the spread of infections. When properly used, there should be no fear of spreading infections from patient to patient or from staff members to the patient, family, and other staff. The caregiver has an important role to play in IPC!

Summary

The topic of infection control and prevention is very important as antibiotics and their "resistance" to organisms is negatively impacting their effectiveness. Handwashing and other measures are key parts of infection control and prevention—whether in the hospital, assisted living, or home or other settings. In your caregiver and advocate role, ask questions and help protect the caregivee/loved one while they are away from home and in a new environment. The resources listed below will help you as you seek to learn more about infection control and prevention.

Resources for You

- The Centers for Disease Control and Prevention (CDC) offers a section called "Cold Versus Flu" to help you know if it is the common cold or the flu: http://www.cdc.gov/flu/about/qa/coldflu.htm
- The CDC also offers the "Handwashing: Clean Hands Save Lives" resource with information about when to wash hands and how to do it effectively: http://www.cdc.gov/handwashing/when-how-handwashing.html
- In addition, the video "Put Your Hands Together" from the CDC also offers information about how vital this action is to infection control: http://www.cdc.gov/CDCTV/handstogether/
- The October 2014 NIH News in Health newsletter featured the article "Cold, Flu, or Allergy? Know the Difference for Best Treatment": http://newsinhealth.nih.gov/issue/oct2014/feature2
- At Flu.gov you can view symptoms, treatment options, vaccine information, and you can enter your zip code to find a vaccination location near you.
- Dartmouth–Hitchcock Medical Center offers a "The Facts: Hand Hygiene" video: https://www.youtube.com/watch?v=txNUEMJUQ7Y

References

Centers for Disease Control and Prevention (CDC). (2015). Nursing Homes and Assisted Living (Long-term Care Facilities [LTCFs]). Retrieved from http://www.cdc.gov/longtermcare/

Centers for Disease Control and Prevention (CDC). (2014a). Hand Hygiene Basics. Retrieved from http://www.cdc.gov/handhygiene/Basics.html

Centers for Disease Control and Prevention (CDC). (2014b). Antibiotic/Antimicrobial Resistance. Retrieved from http://www.cdc.gov/drugresistance/

Centers for Disease Control and Prevention (CDC). (2014c). Show Me the Science—Why Wash Your Hands? Retrieved from http://www.cdc.gov/handwashing/why-handwashing.html

Centers for Disease Control and Prevention (CDC). (2014). New CDC Reports Shows Benefits of Flu Vaccine Last Season But Fewer Than Half of Americans Say They Have Been Vaccinated this Season. Retrieved from http://www.cdc.gov/flu/news/nivw-fewer-vaccinated.htm

Centers for Disease Control and Prevention (CDC). (2013) Preventing Seasonal Flu Illness. Retrieved from http://www.cdc.gov/flu/about/qa/preventing.htm

healthfinder.gov. (2014). Doctors Often Unaware Their Patients Have Catheters. Retrieved from http://www.healthfinder.gov/News/Article.aspx?id=692930&source=govdelivery&utm

MedlinePlus. (n.d.). Germs and Hygiene. Retrieved from http://www.nlm.nih.gov/medlineplus/germsandhygiene.html

–Chapter Eight–

Self-Care of the Caregiver
(Taking Care of Yourself!)

Authors Note: Because I was a registered nurse and made many home visits to home care and hospice patients and families for many years, I thought I knew something about caregiving. This chapter is about what I have learned as a family member caregiver, and what I have gleaned from having the honor of watching family caregivers care for their loved ones. From being a caregiver myself in our home, I have also learned and want to share these tips with you! The bottom line is: There is always more to know. Your efforts to improve care and your caregivee/loved one's life and experiences, and even, perhaps especially, toward end of life, are an opportunity for growth to help your caregivee/loved one's days be the best they can be.

It should go without saying that if you are not caring for yourself, you will not be an effective caregiver. The best thing that caregivers can do for those who depend on them is to take care of themselves. I know this sounds easy—but it is not. Sadly, we sometimes take this for granted and we should not.

Five Things Caregivers Should Stop Doing

1. Don't be the lone caregiver; choose to accept help and stop going it alone, when possible.

2. Sugary foods, alcohol, and cigarettes may feel temporarily good, but they do make you feel worse in the long run. Consider healthier habits to help take care of yourself.

3. Stop listening to "Negative Nellies"—and do not be surprised if they are people, sometimes family members, you least expect it from. Surround yourself with people who are positive and are fun-directed! You need these "Pollyannas" in your life.

4. Stop being afraid to ask for help—make a list of needed activities and consider asking others for assistance. Do not be afraid to delegate! They may not do it perfectly, but it will get done—do not be a perfectionist.

5. Do not neglect your own health. Don't put off your annual doctor visits or other health concerns you may have! You need to be as healthy as you can be—be sure to tell your doctor or nurse practitioner that you are a caregiver!

This is an unusual chapter because this chapter is presented not in paragraphs, but in bullets—so caregivers can read when they need a break and in short pieces or "snippets." The topics are categorized under the headings of "Physical Self-Care Considerations," "Spiritual and Emotional Self-Care Considerations," "Identifying, Preventing, and Relieving Stress," "Identifying When/If It Is No Longer Working at Home," and "Recreational Considerations."

Physical Self-Care Considerations

Get regular exercise when you can. Even if you walk for 10 minutes around your block once or twice a day or park far away in the grocery store parking lot so you get a little walk to and from the car. For example, my husband and I go dancing once a month and I always try to park far away from the entrance of the facility. Consider using the stairs instead of the elevator. It is important to identify what you like to do and to continue doing it—this could be hiking, gardening, or a once a week walking group. Perhaps it helps to have someone you can really talk to and with. Or go to the mall and see the sights while exercising!

Choose to eat healthfully. The "Nutrition for Everyone" site from the Centers for Disease Control and Prevention (CDC) can help guide you: http://www.cdc.gov/nutrition/everyone. Be sure to limit caffeine and alcohol. Getting enough sleep is also important particularly if the caregivee/loved one is up and down during the night. Try to get coverage to allow yourself some uninterrupted sleep.

Spiritual and Emotional Self-Care Considerations

Seek and identify your best spiritual sources of comfort. Make it a habit to pray or practice in your doctrines to help yourself, for a short time every day, even for just five minutes. Spending time with others who also have and value spiritual beliefs can be a great source of comfort. Accept the good intentions of others.

Stay in touch with a family member who lives far away. They know the people/players, and can be more objective as they are not immersed in day-to-day care and dramas, should they arise.

It is difficult to watch those we care for suffer. Even with effective pain and symptom management, this can make the caregiver feel stressed—consider hospice care when care and recovery become unrealistic goals. Let go of the guilt. Realize that we cannot make all things better, and that this is OK.

Maintain relationships and value your long-term friendships. Do not let that important support be a casualty of caregiving—make/take time for yourself!

Identify what you can and cannot change. The Serenity Prayer is commonly recited by caregivers for good reason. You probably know the first part: "God grant me the serenity to accept the things I cannot change; courage to change the things I can; and wisdom to know the difference." Hang one in your house! For example, you cannot change other people's behavior, but you can change your reaction to that behavior. I know this is hard. You can view the full prayer at http:// www.beliefnet.com/Prayers/Protestant/Addiction/Serenity -Prayer.aspx.

Identifying, Preventing, and Relieving Stress

Identify local caregiving support groups and resources in your area. Call your local hospital or ask your doctor for recommendations. This might include transportation to services, your local Agency on Aging, meal deliveries such as "Meals on Wheels,"' home care services, and others.

Make a list of things that can be delegated to others—that they would like to do. This can include taking your caregivee/ loved one on a walk so you have some quiet time for phone calls, driving them to a senior center, or doing your grocery shopping for you—again, so you have some time "off."

Decline requests to do anything that adds to your activities and stress. For example, when your sister-in-law decides that you should host a holiday get-together for 12, just say no!

Accept that no caregiver is perfect—make that okay because caregiving does not lend itself to perfection. Every day is different and may bring different challenges and decisions. (Much like child rearing, which some caregivers may have done.)

Establish a daily routine. This might be that your husband prepares breakfast for your caregivee/loved one and you sleep in a little because you have the evening "get ready for bed" caregiver activities. When possible, this sharing of duties is helpful for avoiding burnout. There is no rule that baths are only in the morning and that there are three big meals prepared and served every day—it is what works for you, your family, and your caregivee/loved one. Give yourself permission to be "outside the box" if it works for you and your caregivee/loved one.

Try to keep your sense of humor. Funny things do happen during caregiving sometimes—it is okay to laugh, and probably very healthy to do so!

Learn all you can about your caregivee/loved one's unique health condition. For example, Alzheimer's, multiple sclerosis, how to care for a urinary catheter—whatever it is—you can learn it and be a better advocate! Learning it helps you to "own" it and be an expert to provide better care. And you can share and teach others from your experience.

Break down big projects into little parts. For example, rather than showering, changing the bed, and washing all the linens in one day, do different tasks on different days—depending on the patient needs. Of course, if the patient is bedridden this might not apply—there would be no shower, but a bed bath. The linens and the bed would need to be changed daily and as needed. In this case, other big tasks could be spread out instead. Sometimes, depending on the situation, you can change the top sheet and the quilt and, more often, for comfort, the pillow cases.

Identifying When/If It Is No Longer Working at Home

You will know when it is not working at home. The burden of care can make the caregiver feel immobilized and overwhelmed and feel they are no longer effective and the caregiver/loved one is not receiving the care they need.

The needs of your caregivee/loved one can no longer be safely met at home. One example is wandering in a confused patient.

If the caregiver is burned out, this might be characterized by a knowledge that they can no longer emotionally or physically provide proper care at home for their caregivee/loved one.

Respite care might also be considered. There are various types of services available including respite care in the home and respite care outside of the home. Consider contacting older adult resources in your community to find out more about respite and related services.

Recreational Considerations

Make time every week to do something that you want to do—such as go to a movie!

Do something for yourself every day—even if it is small. Make one phone call to a friend or take a walk in your garden/yard.

Every four to six weeks have a beauty visit or something similar to look forward to—perhaps a haircut or a manicure.

Leave caregiving when you leave the house. Try and visit with a friend and talk about other things.

When talking with friends, do not make it a stressful recreation of the day—just vent enough that you get loving support and then enjoy their company.

Summary

Caring for the caregiver is an essential part of success for the caregiver and the caregivee/loved one. It is important to care for oneself every day to avoid burnout, which will make you an ineffective caregiver. Attending support groups, saying yes when others offer to help, and planning fun activities and breaks on a regular basis are all healthy behaviors for caregivers. Exercise, good eating habits, and other sound practices help the caregiver be at their optimal level of function.

Take good care of yourself—your caregivee/loved one is depending on it!

Resources for You

- The Centers for Disease Control and Prevention (CDC) offer the "Nutrition for Everyone" page to help guide you in making healthy eating choices: http://www.cdc.gov/nutrition/everyone
- The CDC also offers "Tips for a Safe and Healthy Life": http://www.cdc.gov/family/tips/
- The U.S. Department of Veterans Affairs (VA) offers many

resources in their "VA Caregiver Support" section: http://www.caregiver.va.gov/

- The VA also offers a "Caregiving Self Care" workbook: http://www.caregiver.va.gov/pdfs/Caregiver_Workbook_V3_Module_1.pdf

- The Mayo Clinic has a section on their site devoted to caregiver stress and stress management: http://www.mayoclinic.org/healthy-living/stress-management/in-depth/caregiver-stress/art-20044784

- Medicare.gov has a section for caregivers with resources like "Taking care of yourself" and "What caregiver support is available in my area?": http://www.medicare.gov/campaigns/caregiver/caregiver.html

- The Administration for Community Living (ACL) has a long list of resources specifically for caregivers: http://www.acl.gov/Get_Help/Help_Caregivers/Index.aspx

- The National Institute on Aging offers a guide for Alzheimer's caregivers called "Alzheimer's Caregiving Tips: Caring for Yourself" that includes helpful tips for all caregivers about self-care: https://www.nia.nih.gov/sites/default/files/Alzheimers_Caregiving_Tips_Caring_for_Yourself.pdf

References

beliefnet. (n.d.). Serenity Prayer. Retrieved from http://www.beliefnet.com/Prayers/Protestant/Addiction/Serenity-Prayer.aspx

Chapter Nine

Glossary of Common Health Care Terms

Accreditation: A process that examines various components of health care operations and clinical practice. The achievement of accreditation designates that the organization has gone through the accreditation process and meets predetermined standards as measured by onsite nurses and other survey team "visitors."

Activities of Daily Living (ADL): Basic, usual self-care activities that must be done daily to care for our bodies and overall health. These activities include bathing, dressing, grooming, and toileting including clothing management and hygiene. ADL may also include simple meal preparation or doing laundry. These activities are important indicators because they demonstrate or show the patient's functional status or health care needs.

Advanced Directive: "Advance directives are legal documents that allow you to spell out your decisions about end-of-life care ahead of time" (MedlinePlus, n.d.a) You can include instructions for things like dialysis, breathing machines, feeding tubes, and organ donation (MedlinePlus, n.d.a).

Caregiver: Anyone who provides care or services to or for a patient. According to the National Cancer Institute (2013), "family caregivers may be spouses, partners, children, relatives, or friends who help the patient with activities of daily living and health care needs at home."

Care Plan: A plan of action for care that is developed, delivered, and evaluated by the nurse and other team members. This may also be called the plan of care and varies among organizations. The caregiver and caregivee/loved one should be aware of and have input in this plan of care.

Case Management: A system for overseeing a patient's care usually across health care setings. For example, a nurse or social worker case manager may coordinate care and services from the hospital, to the nursing home, and in the patient's home.

Case Manager: One person who is responsible for the overall care of the patient and use of resources for that care. The case (or care) manager may be a nurse, a social worker, or a therapist.

Catheter: Any rounded or tubular medical device that is inserted into veins, cavities, or other body passages. The purpose of a catheter is to improve or replace function. Examples include a urinary foley catheter in the bladder from which urine drains into a collection bag, suction catheters, and intravenous catheters inserted into the vein which allow for the delivery of fluids.

Chronic Illness: A slow or persistent illness or health problem that must be cared for throughout life. Examples include diabetes, glaucoma, and some chronic lung conditions.

Client: The one who receives care. Also called the patient, customer, or consumer of health care services or products.

Collaboration: The active process of working together and valuing another's input toward reaching patient goals.

CMS: The Centers for Medicare and Medicaid Services. A

part of the U.S. government that administers these health care insurance programs/benefits.

Continuum of Care: A health model meant to track a patient's care over time throughout all healthcare settings they may encounter.

Dementia: Changes in brain function that cause memory loss, confusion, or the loss of ability to function safely and independently.

Diagnosis: The identification of problems or diseases. The singular is diagnosis; the plural is diagnoses.

Dialysis: The process of artificially cleansing the blood when the patient has renal or kidney failure. There are two kinds of dialysis, hemodialysis and peritoneal dialysis.

Dietitian: A member of the health care team who promotes optimal nutrition, based on the patient's individual needs. The dietitian may be called an R.D., a registered dietitian, or an L.D., a licensed dietitian. The dietitian may make home visits or teach the other team members about dietary-related issues such as effective nutrition, meal preparation, and special diets as part of a treatment plan.

Documentation: The writing or electronic entry of clinical notes that contains information needed for communication, legal, and other reasons.

Do Not Resuscitate (DNR): This is a medical order specifically against cardiopulmonary resuscitation (CPR). A patient with this order will not have CPR performed in the case of an emergency.

Edema: Swelling in a particular part of the body. For example, the patient with swelling in the ankles or feet has edema and this should be reported to the nurse.

Enteral Nutrition: Provision of nourishment via a tube inserted into the nose and down to the stomach or through a surgical site through the stomach. A G-tube is an example of enteral nutrition.

G-Tube: Also known as percutaneous endoscopic gastrostomy (PEG) tube. A stomach or gastrostomy tube used to place nutrients into the stomach when the patient cannot safely swallow or eat.

Geriatrics: Specialty services or care related or provided to older adults, related to the process of aging.

Goals: The endpoint of care or the desired results for care. For example, if the goal is to provide safe mobility, everything done should support that goal. The team members, the caregiver, and the caregivee/loved one work to achieve the patient goals.

Health Care Reform: The Patient Protection and Affordable Care Act (PPACA) and Health Care and Education Reconciliation Act of 2010, sometimes jointly called the Affordable Care Act (ACA), expanded coverage for Medicaid and the Children's Health Insurance Program (CHIP) (Medicaid.gov, n.d.).

HIPAA: This stands for the Health Insurance Portability and Accountability Act, which protects patient's medical privacy.

Homebound: A term used in the Medicare home care program that means that the patient cannot leave the home without assistance and that leaving the home is a considerable and taxing effort, which occurs infrequently and lasts for a short duration. Homebound means primarily confined to the home for medical reasons. "Homebound" is one of the admitting criteria for patients admitted to a

Medicare-certified home care program. For this reason, when patients are "no longer homebound," they are discharged from Medicare home health care.

Home Care/Home Health: The provision of a range of health services, products, supplies and equipment to patients in their homes.

Home Health Agency: An organization that provides care to patients in their homes. An agency may or may not be licensed, depending on the state and requirements. Medicare-certified agencies must have a survey or a special review to be certified to accept Medicare patients.

Hospice: A special way of caring for patients and families dealing with a life threatening illness or a limited life expectancy. Hospice tries to make every remaining day the best that it can be. Hospice team members include specially trained hospice volunteers, bereavement counselors, certified nursing assistants (CNAs) or hospice aides, spiritual counselors, nurses, physicians, and other services. Hospice is a philosophy, not a place, but most hospice care is provided at home.

Hyperglycemia: Abnormally high blood sugar or glucose.

Hypertension: Abnormally high blood pressure.

Hypoglycemia: Abnormally low blood sugar or glucose.

Hypotension: Abnormally low blood pressure.

Informed Consent: Because you have the right to know what treatment options are available to you and what disease or condition you have, informed consent refers to the patient being fully informed of this information and the risks involved, and able to understand it, before making decisions about their care. In other words, informed consent must be obtained before treatment can be given and you must have all the information about your disease in order to make any decisions about your healthcare.

Laryngectomy: Surgical removal of the voicebox resulting in the loss of normal speech ability.

LPN or LVN: LPNs and LVNs both work under the guidance of doctors and/or registered nurses. LPN stands for Licensed Practical Nurse and LVN stands for Licensed Vocational Nurse. They typically must complete a 1-year training program to become licensed (Bureau of Labor Statistics, 2014a).

Living Will: This is a type of advanced directive that typically sets out specific rules for what kinds of medical treatments a person would like done if they are in some way incapacitated and no longer able to tell the medical team their decisions.

Medicaid: A health program that is administered at the state level for patients who qualify financially. Medicaid coverage varies by state. Sometimes even the name is different. For example, in California it is called Medi-Cal.

Medical Home: Patient-centered and comprehensive model of primary care that focuses on care coordination.

Medicare: A federal health insurance program for people over age 65, the disabled, or those who have end stage renal disease (ESRD). Medicare is complex and has different parts that cover different services such as inpatient hospitalization (after the Medicare beneficiary pays a deductible), home care, hospice, and other services. Medicare is a medical insurance program, and like all insurance programs there are exclusions, eligibility, and coverage rules. The Centers for Medicare and Medicaid Services (CMS) administer the programs. CMS is a part of the U.S. Department of Health and Human Services (HHS) administration of the government. Part A is hospital insurance while Part B is medical. Part C is advantage plans and Part D is prescription drug coverage.

Medication Reconciliation: CMS calls this the "process of identifying the most accurate list of all medications that the patient is taking, including name, dosage, frequency, and route, by comparing the medical record to an external list of medications obtained from a patient, hospital, or other provider" (2014).

Nurse Practitioner (NP): They have completed a master's or doctorate degree and have advanced clinical training beyond what they achieved in becoming a registered nurse (RN) (American Association of Nurse Practitioners, n.d.).

Occupational Safety and Health Administration (OSHA): The part of the U.S. Government that regulates employee or worker safety. OSHA requires that various standards be maintained related to health care.

Occupational Therapy (OT): The use of therapeutic activity and exercise to help individuals with limitations to function as safely and independently as possible. The OT teaches the use of compensating techniques and assistive devices to improve a person's ability to perform self-care and other ADL such as bathing, meal preparation, etc. Also, OTs address cognitive deficits and instruct in compensation techniques to maximize function.

Outcomes: Outcomes are quantifiable or measurable goals of care. An example of a desirable outcome is that the patient, by a certain date, can name all of their medications, and the time to take them. Outcomes are usually measured across points in time.

Paraplegia: Paralysis or loss of motor ability of the lower extremities or legs.

Palliative Care: Palliative care is treatment of discomfort, symptoms, and stress of serious illness (MedlinePlus, n.d.b). The goal of palliative care is to make patients feel better whether or not they are still receiving curative treatment (MedlinePlus, n.d.c). Hospice care is also one of those special services and is a type of palliative care.

Parenteral Nutrition: The provision of nourishment via an intravenous (IV) route.

Payor: The payor or insurance company financially responsible for the services or care provided to patients. Examples include Medicare or other insurance companies.

Pediatric or Pediatrics: Services or care related to children. Pediatrics is a specialty that involves the development, care, and problems or disease of children and childhood. This includes newborns, infants, toddlers, and all ages of children through adolescence.

Performance Improvement: An ongoing process that seeks to continuously improve patient care, delivery of services, staff education, and other important parts of operations or other parts of an organization. Accreditation standards demand continuous quality improvement. One example could be efforts to improve infection control and prevention in hospitals.

Personal Emergency Response System (PERS): A technology that links the frail or homebound to community resources in the case of a fall or other emergency. PERS usually have a personal help button which when activated, calls for help. To be effective, the PERS personal help button must be worn, carried, or within reach at all times, and used in the event of an emergency.

Pharmacist: Healthcare professionals who work with medications and their safe use. They can be in various settings, including hospitals and skilled nursing facilities; people often do not realize that pharmacists work there, too, and they can ask them questions in these settings as well as at pharmacies.

Physical Therapy (PT): A specialty of the rehabilitation services that focuses on mobility and function of patients due to illness or injury. PTs work with stroke patients, patients with impairments to legs or back, and others who need home exercises or other programs to restore safe mobility and function.

Physician Assistant: Also known as PAs, physician assistants "practice medicine on a team under the supervision of physicians and surgeons. They are formally educated to examine patients, diagnose injuries and illnesses, and provide treatment" (Bureau of Labor Statistics, 2014b).

Polypharmacy: Polypharmacy refers to the use of multiple medications at the same time. It is very common in older adults. This can be appropriate, but should be continually reviewed.

Quadriplegia: Paralysis or loss of motor ability of all upper and lower extremities, both arms and legs. This is also called tetraplegia.

Registered Nurse: "Registered nurses (RNs) provide and coordinate patient care, educate patients and the public about various health conditions, and provide advice and emotional support to patients and their family members"

(Bureau of Labor Statistics, 2015). Registered nurses must have a bachelor's or associate's degree and be licensed in the state(s) in which they practice.

Rehabilitation: The term used to describe the care and efforts of team members to restore function and mobility after illness or injury. Members of the rehabilitation team include the physical therapist, occupational therapist, and speech-language pathologist.

Respiratory Therapy: The respiratory therapist is a specialist usually involved with patients who need oxygen or have other respiratory problems or illnesses.

Respite Care: Short-term care meant to provide temporary relief to caregivers.

Social Work Services (SWS): Social work services, also called medical social services (MSS), are valuable services to patients and their families for a number of reasons. The social worker or medical social worker (MSW) may be involved when there are problems that prevent the plan of care from being implemented. For example, a social worker might be involved if the patient has diabetes and cannot afford food or insulin, or if there are family or other problems that are causing the patient not to improve or to be in unsafe conditions. A social worker at the hospital may be involved in your caregivee/loved one's discharge from the hospital back to home or to another care setting. Medical social workers (MSWs) provide assistance to patients and their families in identifying financial and community resources. They may also provide counseling or bereavement services.

Speech-Language Pathology (SLP): The speech-language pathologist or speech therapist is involved primarily with patients who have swallowing or communication problems due to surgery or other problems such as a stroke.

Standard Precautions: "Minimum infection prevention practices that apply to all patient care, regardless of suspected or confirmed infection status of the patient, in any setting where healthcare is delivered" (Centers for Disease Control and Prevention [CDC], 2015).

Supervisory Visit: Supervision is a standard practice in home and hospice care and assists in assuring quality of care for patients. A registered nurse (RN) is required to provide supervision of licensed practical nurses (LPN) and home health aides. These supervisory visits are to assess the overall quality of care and may be done while the LPN or aide is present or may occur when they are not there.

Technician: A technician is someone in a hospital or clinic setting who will analyze tests, including body fluids and tissue samples. Depending on the setting, they may have either a bachelor's or associate's degree, and they may or may not have to be licensed depending on the state they practice in. This includes a medical technician, a lab technician, or a patient care technician.

Tracheostomy: Surgical creation of an opening in the skin to the trachea, the breathing tube.

Venipuncture: A puncture into the vein to draw blood. The nurse or lab technician obtains blood through venipuncture for laboratory analysis.

References

American Association of Nurse Practitioners. (n.d.). What's an NP? Retrieved from http://www.aanp.org/all-about-nps/what-is-an-np

Centers for Medicare and Medicaid (CMS). (2014). Eligible Professional Meaningful Use Menu Set Measures Measure 6 of 9. Retrieved from http://www.cms.gov/Regulations-and-Guidance/Legislation/EHR IncentivePrograms/downloads/7_Medication_Reconciliation.pdf

Bureau of Labor Statistics. (2015). Registered Nurses. Retrieved from http://www.bls.gov/ooh/healthcare/registered-nurses.htm

Bureau of Labor Statistics. (2014a). Licensed Practical and Licensed Vocational Nurses. Retrieved from http://www.bls.gov/ooh/healthcare/licensed-practical-and-licensed-vocational-nurses.htm

Bureau of Labor Statistics. (2014b). Physician Assistants. Retrieved from http://www.bls.gov/ooh/healthcare/physician-assistants.htm

Centers for Disease Control and Prevention. (2015). Guide to Infection Prevention for Outpatient Settings: Minimum Expectations for Safe Care. Retrieved from http://www.cdc.gov/HAI/settings/outpatient/outpatient-care-gl-standard-precautions.html

Medicaid.gov. (n.d.). Affordable Care Act. Retrieved from http://medicaid.gov/affordablecareact/affordable-care-act.html

MedlinePlus. (n.d.a). Advance Directives. Retrieved from http://www.nlm.nih.gov/medlineplus/advancedirectives.html

MedlinePlus. (n.d.b). Palliative Care. Retrieved from http://www.nlm.nih.gov/medlineplus/palliativecare.html

MedlinePlus. (n.d.c). What is palliative care? Retrieved from http://www.nlm.nih.gov/medlineplus/ency/patientinstructions/000536.htm

National Cancer Institute. (2013). Family Caregivers in Cancer. Retrieved from http://www.cancer.gov/cancertopics/pdq/supportivecare/caregivers/patient/page1

Chapter Ten

Directory of Further Resources

This section contains further resources, often for more big-picture information if you are interested in a specific area. Some of these resources are books or other media for more information while others are interesting reads and information related to overall health care and caregiving.

Caregiver Health

Womenshealth.gov offers a "Caregiver stress fact sheet" with information about who are the most common caregivers, how stress from caregiving can affect your health, and what to do if you need a break from caregiving: http://www.womens health.gov/publications/our-publications/fact-sheet/caregiver stress.html?from=AtoZ

The U.S. Department of Veterans Affairs offers a VA Caregiver Support resource page that includes information specific to caregivers about staying organized, tips, checklists, and caring for yourself: http://www.caregiver.va.gov/

KidsHealth offers a resource for caregivers called "Taking Care of You: Support for Caregivers": http://kidshealth.org/ parent/system/ill/caregivers.html

The National Institute on Aging's AgePage has a resource called "Long-Distance Caregiving—Getting Started" to help you if you are not able to be a caregiver from the home

of the caregivee/loved one: http://www.nia.nih.gov/health/
publication/long-distance-caregiving-getting-started

Family Caregiver Alliance's guide to "Taking Care of YOU:
Self-Care for Family Caregivers": https://www
.caregiver.org/taking-care-you-self-care-family-caregivers

Children

Make-A-Wish grants wishes to children facing life-
threatening medical conditions: http://wish.org/about-us

The Complex Child E-Magazine offers information for caregivers caring for children with special needs: http://www
.complexchild.com/

The United Mitochondrial Disease Foundation offers a list
of Mitochondrial Related Organizations: http://www.umdf
.org/site/c.jtJWJaMMIsE/b.4090419/k.5FDE/Mitochondrial_
Related_Organizations.htm

The National Alliance for Caregiving and AARP offer "The
Caregivers of Children: A Focused Look at Those Caring
for A Child with Special Needs Under the Age of 18," which
includes information about caregivers who specifically care
for children: http://assets.aarp.org/rgcenter/il/caregiving_09_
children.pdf

The U.S. Department of Education has a section on their
site with resources on "My Child's Special Needs": http://
www2.ed.gov/parents/needs/speced/edpicks.jhtml

The University of Michigan Health System offers information about "Children with Chronic Conditions" including
descriptions of what constitutes a chronic condition: http://
www.med.umich.edu/yourchild/topics/chronic.htm

The Centers for Disease Control and Prevention (CDC) has a site with information about diseases and conditions that might affect infants and toddlers: http://www.cdc.gov/parents/infants/diseases_conditions.html

MedlinePlus also offers information on common infant and newborn conditions: http://www.nlm.nih.gov/medlineplus/commoninfantandnewbornproblems.html

The American Psychological Association has an information page for parent caregivers called "When your child is diagnosed with chronic illness: How to cope": http://www.apa.org/helpcenter/chronic-illness-child.aspx

Chronic Conditions

The Centers for Disease Control and Prevention (CDC) offer an overview of chronic diseases: http://www.cdc.gov/chronicdisease/overview/

The National Diabetes Education Program offers information for people with diabetes and their caregivers including resources on caring for people with diabetes and helping to control your diabetes: http://www.ndep.nih.gov/

The National Heart, Lung, and Blood Institute offers information about conditions related to heart, lung, and blood diseases including coronary heart disease, Chronic Obstructive Pulmonary Disease (COPD), and anemia: http://www.nhlbi.nih.gov/

The Agency for Healthcare Research and Quality (AHRQ) provides information about care coordination, which "involves deliberately organizing patient care activities and sharing information among all of the participants concerned with a patient's care to achieve safer and more effective care": www.ahrq.gov/professionals/prevention-chronic-care/improve/coordination/

The American Medical Association and the Centers for Disease Control (CDC) have partnered for a Prevent Diabetes STAT campaign, which stands for Screen, Test, Act Today to help recognize prediabetes and work toward preventing new cases of diabetes: http://www.ama-assn.org/sub/prevent-diabetes-stat/index.html?utm_source=(direct)&utm_medium=(none)&utm_term=vanity&utm_content=prediabetes_stat&utm_campaign=partnership

Eating Healthy

Let's Move offers information about eating healthy and staying active: http://www.letsmove.gov/eat-healthy

The President's Council on Fitness, Sports & Nutrition offers "Eight Healthy Eating Goals": http://www.fitness.gov/eat-healthy/how-to-eat-healthy/

The Centers for Disease Control and Prevention (CDC) offers a resource for finding healthy recipes: http://www.cdc.gov/healthyweight/healthy_eating/recipes.html

The Centers for Disease Control and Prevention (CDC) also offer a Nutrition for Everyone page with information about what to eat and how much of each food group and different vitamins you need: http://www.cdc.gov/nutrition/everyone/

Emergency Preparedness

The Centers for Disease Control and Prevention's (CDC) emergency preparedness and response page provides up-to-date information about natural disasters, current outbreaks of disease, and more: http://emergency.cdc.gov/

Five Days at Memorial: Life and Death in a Storm-Ravaged Hospital is a book about one hospital's experience during Hurricane Katrina by Sheri Fink.

If you own pets, Ready.gov also has a section for preparing to care for your pets during an emergency: http://www.ready.gov/caring-animals

End of Life

A good book about living life to the fullest, especially in our personal relationships, is *The Four Things That Matter Most: A Book About Living* by Ira Byock.

The National Institute on Aging (NIA) has a page to help with making end-of-life decisions called "End of Life: Helping With Comfort and Care": http://www.nia.nih.gov/health/publication/end-life-helping-comfort-and-care/planning-end-life-care-decisions

MedlinePlus offers information about advance directives: http://www.nlm.nih.gov/medlineplus/advancedirectives.html

MedlinePlus also has information about what palliative care is: http://www.nlm.nih.gov/medlineplus/palliativecare.html

AARP has a "Caregiving Resource Center" with information about end of life, end-of-life discussions, and finding a provider near you: http://www.aarp.org/home-family/caregiving/end-of-life.html

Cancer Care offers a resource dealing with end of life called "Caregiving at the End of Life": http://www.cancercare.org/publications/63-caregiving_at_the_end_of_life

The National Cancer Institute offers many end-of-life resources, including "Preparing for the End of Life" (http://www.cancer.gov/cancertopics/coping/end-of-life), "Palliative Care in Cancer" (http://www.cancer.gov/cancertopics/advanced-cancer/care-choices/palliative-care-fact-sheet), and "Last Days of Life" (http://www.cancer.gov/cancertopics/pdq/supportivecare/lasthours/patient/page1/AllPages/Print).

NIHSeniorHealth has a resource for those facing the end of life called "Preparing For The End of Life" that includes how to define the end of life and addressing symptoms like pain: http://nihseniorhealth.gov/endoflife/preparingfortheendoflife/01.html

Aging with Dignity is an organization that offers many resources for those facing the end of life, including the "Five Wishes," a popular living will option that is legally recognized in 42 states. It is available in 28 languages: https://www.agingwithdignity.org/five-wishes.php

Falls

NIHSeniorHealth offers a resource called "Falls and Older Adults" that includes tips for older adults about how to get up from a fall and information about emergency response devices: http://nihseniorhealth.gov/falls/ifyoufall/01.html.

The Centers for Disease Control and Prevention (CDC) have a section of their site devoted to "Hip Fractures Among

Older Adults" that discusses who is at risk and how you can help prevent them: http://www.cdc.gov/homeandrecreational safety/falls/adulthipfx.html

Health Care Reform

Healthfinder.gov offers information about health care reform, including explanations of preventative services: http://www .healthfinder.gov/HealthCareReform/

The Robert Wood Johnson Foundation offers the "Talk-HealthInsurance to Me" site to help answer questions about the recent changes to health insurance: http://talkhealth insurancetome.org/

Infection Control

The Doctors' Plague: Germs, Childbed Fever, and the Strange Story of Ignac Semmelweis by Sherwin Nuland is a non-fiction book about the importance of infection control told through the story of one doctor who was on a mission to stop the spread of disease from doctors themselves.

The Great Influenza: The Story of the Deadliest Pandemic in History by John M. Barry is a non-fiction book that tells the story of the flu epidemic that killed more than 100 million people during WWI.

The Centers for Disease Control and Prevention (CDC) offers information about the seasonal flu vaccine and who should and should not be vaccinated (http://www.cdc.gov/flu/ protect/keyfacts.htm) as well as information about how long germs can live on surfaces (http://www.cdc.gov/flu/about/qa/ preventing.htm) and how long you should remain home, and away from anyone with a weakened immune system, while you have symptoms (http://www.cdc.gov/flu/takingcare.htm).

The CDC also has information available about healthcare-associated infections (HAIs) (http://www.cdc.gov/hai/) and "Hand Hygiene in Healthcare Settings" (http://www.cdc.gov/HandHygiene/index.html).

The Agency for Healthcare Research and Quality (AHRQ) also has information about HAIs: http://www.psnet.ahrq.gov/primer.aspx?primerID=7

MedlinePlus has a useful definition of infection control available: http://www.nlm.nih.gov/medlineplus/infectioncontrol.html

The Association for Professionals in Infection Control and Epidemiology (APIC) has a page of information available about home care specifically: http://www.apic.org/About-APIC/Membership-sections/Home-Care

The Minnesota Department of Health provides a useful set of "Infection Prevention and Control Guidelines": http://www.health.state.mn.us/divs/idepc/dtopics/infectioncontrol/guidelines.html

The United States Environmental Protection Agency (EPA) provides information about "Protecting Yourself from Bed Bugs in Public Places": http://www2.epa.gov/bedbugs/protecting-yourself-bed-bugs-public-places

Kidney Care

The Coalition for Supportive Care of Kidney Patients (CSCKP) offers resources and information to help support care for kidney patients: http://www.kidneysupportivecare.org/Home.aspx

Medicare

Medicare.gov is the official site for Medicare and can help you determine if a test, item, or service is covered and where to find a doctor, provider, or hospital. They also offer resources like the "Medicare and Home Health Care" booklet (https://www.medicare.gov/Pubs/pdf/10969.pdf) and "Medicare & You 2015" (http://www.medicare.gov/Pubs/pdf/10050 .pdf).

Medications and Medication Assistance

National Jewish Health offers a resource about "What You Need to Know When Taking Anticoagulant Medicine": http://www.nationaljewish.org/NJH/media/pdf/MF-Taking-Anticoagulation-Medicine.pdf?ext=.pdf

The Partnership for Prescription Assistance offers information about patient assistance programs for prescriptions and a tool for finding a clinic near you: https://www.pparx.org/ or 1-888-477-2669

NeedyMeds is a site to help you find financial assistance for medicine: NeedyMeds.com or 1-800-503-6897

Rx Outreach helps provide affordable medications: www .rxoutreach.com or 1-800-769-3880

The Agency for Healthcare Research and Quality (AHRQ) has a guide called "Blood Thinner Pills: Your Guide to Using Them Safely": http://www.ahrq.gov/patients-consumers/ diagnosis-treatment/treatments/btpills/btpills.html

The U.S. Food and Drug Administration (FDA) has a consumer section of their site with information about recent updates as well as a section of audience-specific information for groups including women, patient advocates, seniors, and parents: http://www.fda.gov/ForConsumers/

Older Adult Health

Healthfinder.gov has information about specific conditions, health recommendations by age, and information about health care reform.

The National Institute on Aging offers research and information on aging, particularly Alzheimer's Disease: http://www.nia.nih.gov/

The American Geriatrics Society offers information about older adults and conditions they may face through their Health in Aging Foundation: http://www.healthinaging foundation.org/

Familydoctor.org offers information for people of all ages on topics like health insurance, medications, self-care, and working with your doctor.

The National Institute on Aging's AgePage offers a resource called "Hospital Hints" to prepare you for a hospital visit, including what to bring, what to leave at home, and safety tips while in the hospital: http://www.nia.nih.gov/health/publication/hospital-hints

The National Institute on Aging's AgePage also offers a resource on "Nursing Homes: Making the Right Choice": http://www.nia.nih.gov/health/publication/nursing-homes

The Centers for Disease Control and Prevention's (CDC) website offers many resources with reliable and up-to-date health information about conditions such as the flu, travelling safely, and emergency preparedness: www.cdc.gov

The Eldercare Locator from the Department of Health and Human Services offers a search tool for finding help for your caregivee/loved one based on the problem they may be facing, like long term care needs or nutrition, and your location: eldercare.gov or call 1-800-677-1116

HealthinAging.org offers resources for older adults and their caregivers including resources on caring from a distance and medication use in older adults.

The Administration on Aging (AoA) offers resources for caregivers in general as well as specific information about conditions and helping your caregivee/loved one if they have a disability: http://aoa.gov/

LongTermCare.gov provides information about what long-term care is, who might need it, considerations for the LGBT community, Alzheimer's considerations, and how to find local providers: http://longtermcare.gov/the-basics/

The Health Resources and Services Administration (HRSA) offers information about health care on their website including a search tool to find a health center near you: http://www.hrsa.gov/

The Agency for Healthcare Research and Quality (AHRQ) offers a resource called "20 Tips to Help Prevent Medical Errors" to help you understand what medical errors are and what you can do to help prevent them: http://www.ahrq.gov/patients-consumers/care-planning/errors/20tips/20tips.pdf

The National Cancer Institute offers information on their website including explanations of common cancer types http://www.cancer.gov/

Next Step in Care has a page of information about what durable medical equipment is for family caregivers: http://

www.nextstepincare.org/Caregiver_Home/Durable_
Medical_Equipment/?tr=y&auid=15333472

U.S. Department of Health & Human Services offers information on multiple chronic conditions: http://www.hhs
.gov/ash/initiatives/mcc/

The U.S. Department of Health & Human Services provides resources on their website on a wide range of topics and links to other government health-related sites: HHS.gov

The Institute for Healthcare Improvement offers information on topics like catheter-associated urinary tract infections, pressure ulcers, and surgical site infections: http://www.ihi
.org/

Pain Management

MedlinePlus offers a resource on "Post surgical pain treatment—adults": http://www.nlm.nih.gov/medlineplus/
ency/patientinstructions/000406.htm

Patient Consent

The Immortal Life of Henrietta Lacks by Rebecca Skloot is a non-fiction book about the amazing story of how a woman's cells were taken, without her knowledge or consent, and used in medical research. This true story addresses what we now value about privacy, permissions, and more.

Safety

The Agency for Healthcare Research and Quality (AHRQ) offers a collection of information about patient safety in their Patient Safety Network section: http://psnet.ahrq.gov/

The Agency for Healthcare Research and Quality (AHRQ) also has a booklet available called "Taking Care of Myself: A Guide for When I Leave the Hospital": http://www.ahrq.gov/patients-consumers/diagnosis-treatment/hospitals-clinics/goinghome/index.html

Medicare.gov offers a "Guide to Choosing a Hospital": http://www.medicare.gov/Publications/Pubs/pdf/10181.pdf

The National Patient Safety Foundation offers a section of resources for patients and their families with guides like "Getting the Right Diagnosis" and "From Hospital to Home": http://www.npsf.org/?page=patientsandfamilies

Smoking Cessation

The U.S. Department of Health and Human Services offers the "Want to Quit Smoking? We Can Help!" resource: http://www.hhs.gov/blog/2015/03/24/want-quit-smoking-we-can-help.html?utm_campaign=032415_hhs_blog_smoke free&utm_medium=email&utm_source=hhs_blog_updates &utm_content=032415_hhs_blog_smokefree_titlelink

Many health-related apps can be downloaded to your smartphone, like the "SinceiQuit" app for iPhones: https://itunes.apple.com/us/app/since-iquit/id334825691?mt=8

Spanish Language Resources

The National Institute on Aging offers many Spanish resources: http://www.nia.nih.gov/espanol

The National Institute on Aging's AgePage offers a resource called "Hospital Hints" to prepare you for a hospital visit, including what to bring, what to leave at home, and safety tips while in the hospital: http://www.nia.nih.gov/espanol/publicaciones/consejos-cuando-debe-ir-al-hospital

The Centers for Disease Control and Prevention's (CDC) website offers many resources with reliable and up-to-date health information about conditions such as the flu, travelling safely, and emergency preparedness: http://www.cdc.gov/spanish/

The National Diabetes Education Program offers information for people with diabetes and their caregivers including resources on caring for people with diabetes and helping to control your diabetes: http://www.ndep.nih.gov/i-have-diabetes/TengoDiabetes.aspx

The Robert Wood Johnson Foundation offers the Talk-HealthInsurance to me site to help answer questions about the recent changes to health insurance: http://talkhealth insurancetome.org/?lang=es

Next Step in Care has a page of information about what durable medical equipment is for family caregivers: http://www.nextstepincare.org/uploads/File/Guides/Durable_Medical_Equipment/Durable_Medical_Equipment_Spanish.pdf

The Agency for Healthcare Research and Quality (AHRQ) has a guide called "Blood Thinner Pills: Your

Guide to Using Them Safely": http://www.ahrq.gov/patients-consumers/diagnosis-treatment/treatments/btpills/btpills.html

Spiritual Care

The HealthCare Chaplaincy Network is a nonprofit dedicated to helping people find comfort and meaning when facing illness: http://www.healthcarechaplaincy.org/

Veterans

The U.S. Department of Veterans Affairs (VA) offers many resources for veterans on their site including information about health benefits, finding hospitals, and health care reform: http://va.gov/

The VA also offers resources for dealing with posttraumatic stress disorder (PTSD): http://www.ptsd.va.gov/

We Honor Veterans provides information for veterans about special care considerations and veteran organizations: http://www.wehonorveterans.org/

The Wounded Warrior Project offers information about supporting wounded veterans: http://www.woundedwarrior-project.org/

Paralyzed Veterans of America offers information about getting support for veterans who are paralyzed: http://www.pva.org/site/c.ajIRK9NJLcJ2E/b.6349695/k.97DA/Get_Support.htm

We Honor Veterans is an organization that aims to help veterans at the end of life through hospice partnerships and programs like the veteran-to-veteran volunteers, which matches veteran volunteers to veterans who are at the end of life: http://www.wehonorveterans.org./

Part Two

Special Patient Populations
Care Information by Problem

ALZHEIMER'S DISEASE AND DEMENTIA CARE

I. Introduction: Alzheimer's disease is a dementia or progressive decline in one's cognition and memory. Cognition refers to conscious mental abilities, such as thinking, understanding, learning, and remembering. Caregivee/loved ones with Alzheimer's disease have confusion, increasing memory loss, disorientation, the loss of problem solving abilities, and, sadly, a gradual deterioration in the ability to function and care for themselves. There can be other causes of dementia and dementia symptoms. Because of this, a thorough evaluation and diagnostic work-up should be done before there is a diagnosis of dementia. For example, normal pressure hydrocephalus (NPH) can also cause dementia and the dementia from NPH is potentially reversible. Depression, psychosis, vitamin deficiencies, thyroid disease, medications and their interactions/side effects, and other medical problems should also be investigated. This "befuddlement" or new mental confusion can also be a result of a change in environment and other factors, such as an acute infection, like a urinary tract infection. It is important to note that if your caregivee/loved one have a sudden or "new" onset of confusion that comes on quickly, it needs to be brought to the attention of the physician because dementia is not "sudden." It is usually progressive and develops over time.

Research reported by the National Institute on Aging suggests that as many as 5 million Americans have Alzheimer's disease, although estimates about that number vary (National

Institute on Aging, n.d.). This disease usually occurs after age 65, and it is the most common cause of dementia in older people. For more information about Alzheimer's disease visit: www.nia.nih.gov/alzheimers. You will also find more Alzheimer's-specific resources listed at the end of this chapter.

You may also refer to other chapters in this book such as: "Bedbound Care (Care of the Immobilized or Bedridden Patient)," "Stroke Care (Cerebrovascular Accident)," "End-of-Life Care," "Older Adult Care," and Chapter Six: Safety in the Home: The Most Frequent Health Care Setting of Choice!

2. General Information: The statistics above let you know that you are not alone as a caregiver in this situation. The stress of caring for someone with this illness is tremendous. Alzheimer's disease is progressive, meaning that your caregivee/loved one's needs will increase as time goes on. Alzheimer's disease can progress very slowly for a long time. For this reason, one of the main difficulties of caring for someone with Alzheimer's disease and other dementias is the stress on the caregiver(s). It is very important that the caregiver develop good self-care habits. We encourage you to read Chapter Eight: Self-Care of the Caregiver (Taking Care of Yourself!). As a caregiver of someone with Alzheimer's or dementia, you may begin to feel that you have lost control of your life, or of the life that you once knew. This is especially true if your caregivee/loved one is a spouse or life partner or other close relative. You may experience grieving. The support resources listed at the end of this chapter provide specialized information, designed specifically for caregivers of caregivee/loved ones who have Alzheimer's disease or dementia.

Safety, health maintenance, prevention of wandering, and general support are the main concerns for the caregivers of a confused or disoriented caregivee/loved one. The caregivee/loved one may forget to eat, may have difficulty sleeping, and/or have other disruptions in their daily routines. They may need to be reminded to eat, drink, or urinate. They may develop bizarre or unsafe behaviors and have other personality changes. Because individuals lose the ability to care for themselves over time, they eventually lose the ability to feed and toilet themselves.

3. General Goals for Care: The bottom line goal is twofold and includes both you and your caregivee/loved one. Both goals are equally important!

a. The goal for your caregivee/loved one is that they are safe and comfortable; have nutritious meals; have plenty to drink; to gain as much enjoyment out of life as possible; and experience minimal discomfort, pain, and anxiety. Alzheimer's and dementia caregivee/loved ones need plenty of rest and, perhaps most importantly, they need consistency in their daily activities. As much as possible, they should be allowed to go at their own pace and may need to be gently reoriented to their surroundings throughout the day. You will want to always be sure that your caregivee/loved one is urinating enough and that their urine color is not too dark in color. These caregivee/loved ones should be having regular bowel movements; this is especially important if they are on pain medication. Please call your doctor or clinic if your caregivee/loved one goes more than three days without a bowel movement! Comfort is always a goal for any caregivee/loved one, regardless of their illness. Later in this chapter you will find more specific information about ways to help the caregivee/loved one with Alzheimer's or dementia be more comfortable.

b. It is very important that you, as caregiver, maintain a sense of control over your life. The caregivee/loved one with Alzheimer's or dementia can become very dependent upon one person (you!) for care. This is because they depend upon consistency in order to feel safe. As the caregiver, you may benefit from the support resources listed at the end of this chapter. And we strongly encourage you to seek local resources, perhaps at churches or community centers near you. Patience and kindness from you toward your caregivee/loved one and from you toward yourself is in order here. You may need to find a way to take time out from the repetition of caring for the caregivee/loved one who is experiencing ongoing memory loss with personality and behavior changes.

4. Personal Care Considerations: Your caregivee/loved one needs to feel safe and comfortable in their environment. How you communicate with your caregivee/loved one is key to this. A caregivee/loved one with Alzheimer's or dementia needs a calm and quiet environment. Communication with them should always be supportive, positive, and encouraging. In addition, sometimes written communication using a large font with easy-to-read, block print can be better processed by the individual with Alzheimer's disease than spoken language. They do better with consistency, meaning meals at the same time every day and baths or daily grooming routines at the same time and in the same manner every day. Changes in routine, sudden changes in the environment, and loud noises can be disruptive and/or frightening to these caregivee/loved ones. When you are communicating with your caregivee/

loved one, a quiet tone and patience will go a long way. You may need to repeat your guidance or instructions to them, even for activities that were always routine. In all activities with these caregivee/loved ones, explain what you are going to do and what you are doing as you do it. Short and concise instructions are the most effective. Often caregivee/loved ones with Alzheimer's or dementia are more alert earlier in the day. Their memory and abilities may decline in the afternoon and evening. This is very common and is referred to as "sundowning."

Generally, a high calorie diet can help prevent weight loss. Use of simple, one-step instructions to encourage food intake is helpful to your caregivee/loved one. For example, "Put the food on your fork. Put the food in your mouth. Chew. Swallow." This should be done without rushing the caregivee/loved one. Some people with Alzheimer's disease/dementia may find it easier to eat finger foods. Speak with your doctor, nurse, or health care team if your caregivee/loved one has trouble swallowing or has a diminished appetite.

Your caregivee/loved one may, over time, develop a fear of water. They may fear and/or resist showering or bathing. Calm, quiet encouragement and positive reassurance, without rushing, is often helpful when encountering resistance in these areas. Sometimes distracting your caregivee/loved one with a story or fond memory will help them move forward with the task at hand. Deferring the bath or shower to another time may be a good idea. Perhaps the caregivee/loved one will let another person perform a task and, if that is the case, use that "gift" to take a bit of time for yourself! The bathing process may be quite scary for some people with Alzheimer's disease or dementia; they may be cold and frightened when undressed. Allow the caregivee/loved one to do as much personal and self-care as possible. It is good to remember that Alzheimer's disease or dementia caregivee/loved ones do best with consistent routines. You may need to "cue" your caregivee/loved one for the order of the desired activities. If your caregivee/loved one is incontinent, regular "toileting" (offering the opportunity to use the toilet) may serve as a reminder and may prevent "accidents." It is important to change their undergarments or incontinent pads/briefs whenever they become soiled and to keep their skin as clean and dry as possible. Keep in mind that wet skin is more prone to breakdown. You will want to report any red areas that do not go away to the doctor, nurse, or health care team.

A clean, fresh mouth helps a caregivee/loved one feel comfortable. It helps them eat and digest their food properly, and a clean mouth will head off any mouth problems at an early stage. Sometimes, those suffering from Alzheimer's disease or dementia may resist mouth care. Tasks such as brushing their teeth or allowing their dentures to be cleaned still need to be done daily. If gentle coaxing doesn't work, perhaps asking or even designating this task to another family member may be a good idea. Try to do it at the same time every day. If you see any mouth sores or a white coating on the tongue, and/or if your caregivee/loved one has any difficulty swallowing, let your doctor, nurse, or health care team know right away.

5. Safety Considerations: Always remember safety first when helping your caregivee/loved one. Alzheimer's disease or dementia caregivee/loved ones often forget what was once considered second-nature safety tasks. The changes we are describing here usually happen gradually. We encourage you to be proactive; that is, to anticipate safety needs before an accident or incident occurs. It is always better (and easier!) to prevent a problem than to address a bigger problem after it occurs. And please, if your loved one is still driving, this is a major safety issue! Ask your doctor for guidance in this area.

Safety will be especially important in the kitchen and in the bathroom. Scan *all* areas of your house for any objects that could cause injury, including items that could be swallowed and cause choking.

In the kitchen, your caregivee/loved one may need to be protected from burning themselves or their environment. Consider all types of stoves and ovens, including microwave ovens, as a potential hazard. Stoves and ovens may need to be disconnected. Your caregivee/loved one with Alzheimer's or dementia may be unable to tell if the kitchen, bath, or shower water temperature is too hot or too cold. They can sometimes become fearful of mirrors because they do not recognize the image that they are seeing. This can cause them to become agitated, and agitation can quickly become a safety concern.

Sometimes, caregivee/loved ones who have Alzheimer's disease or dementia "wander away." They may become disoriented and "lost" in the home or they may wander outside and become disoriented and lost. They may be unable to tell if the weather is dangerously hot or cold. They may lose the ability to find their way home or the ability to ask for help. They might not remember how to use a telephone and they might not remember their address. It's a good idea to keep an identification card on the caregivee/loved one with Alzheimer's disease or dementia and keep the doors locked. Use child proof locks on doors and cabinets as needed. You may also consider a bracelet or some other type of identification with an emergency number to keep on your caregivee/loved one at all times. In addition, consider having the caregivee/loved one wear a bracelet with global positioning (GPS) chips for those at risk for wandering. These personal transmitters are usually worn at all times.

Readers are also encouraged to refer to Chapter Six: Safety in the Home: The Most Frequent Health Care Setting of Choice!

6. When to Call the Doctor, Nurse, or Care Team: These are only possible examples and NOT an inclusive list. Please remember that calling *before* a situation becomes a bigger problem is always best. It's better to catch problems when they are relatively small. It is much harder to address "big" problems.

- Caregivee/loved one shows a change in their behavior. For example, they become agitated, angry, frightened, or are showing other signs of obvious distress.
- Caregivee/loved one sees things or people who are not there.
- Caregivee/loved one hears sounds or voices that are not real.
- Caregivee/loved one begins wandering.
- Caregivee/loved one cannot fall asleep or wakes up frequently during the night.
- Caregivee/loved one has distressful nausea or nausea that won't go away, with or without vomiting.
- Caregivee/loved one has stopped eating or drinking or has difficulty swallowing.
- Caregivee/loved one has a change in how they urinate. Perhaps they cannot urinate or they are urinating much more

frequently than usual, but only producing small amounts of urine. Perhaps their urine has changed color, is very dark, and/or has a strong odor. Increased confusion can be an early sign of a urinary tract or other infection.

- Caregivee/loved one has had a change in their bowel movements or has stopped having bowel movements for more than three days, even if they are not eating very much.
- Caregivee/loved ones become incontinent of urine or stool or both.
- Caregivee/loved one has fallen.
- Caregivee/loved one has unexplained bruising or larger bruises than you would normally expect.
- Caregivee/loved one has a sudden or high fever.
- Caregivee/loved one complains of pain.
- Caregivee/loved one has white spots or a white coating on their tongue, or any other kind of mouth sore. This may or may not be accompanied by difficulty swallowing.
- Any other change, complication, or concern that you or the caregivee/loved one may have. When in doubt, call!

These are examples only. Your caregivee/loved one might relay to you changes or concerns that vary from those listed here and those concerns should be addressed with your care team.

7. Comfort Considerations: Comfort for your caregivee/loved one can mean physical, mental, spiritual, or any combination of those kinds of comfort. As a caregiver, providing comfort for your caregivee/loved one sometimes means "the small things." Small things are sometimes easily overlooked. Having regular bowel movements may seem like a small thing, but it is actually a very large part of caregivee/loved one comfort. If your caregivee/loved one is on any pain medication, they can and, in many cases, do cause constipation. You may need to keep track of their bowel movements to prevent constipation.

In regards to physical discomfort, changing positions or a gentle back rub and/or massage may help. A heating pad and/or cold/ice compress should not be used and can be dangerous to a caregivee/loved one with Alzheimer's disease or dementia.

Sometimes, the Alzheimer's disease or dementia caregivee/loved one can become agitated for no apparent reason. Distraction can ease the discomfort that this mental agitation causes. Some caregivee/loved ones respond to, and may become very attached to, a stuffed animal, baby doll, or soft blanket or quilt (this does not mean the caregivee/loved one is to be treated as a child, they should be respected at all times). Playing CDs of the caregivee/loved one's favorite music, watching a favorite TV show or movie, playing cards, or photo sharing are some activities you may like to try. Spending time with a pet can be a wonderful, calming therapy. A visit to a place that was once meaningful, such as their spiritual center, the ocean, or the mountains may be a calming comfort measure. It is important to remember that caregivee/loved ones with Alzheimer's disease or dementia respond differently to different types of comfort measures. For example, watching TV or going for a drive may be calming for some, but may cause others to become agitated or overly stimulated. You will learn over time and by "trial and error" what works best for you and your caregivee/loved one. Sometimes your caregivee/loved one may reject you as their caregiver. Please don't take this personally! This is just one of the ways that Alzheimer's disease or dementia deeply affects and disrupts the life of the caregiver. If this happens, allow yourself restful time away and, whenever possible, do something nice for yourself.

Respect the caregivee/loved one's privacy and dignity at all times.

8. Special Considerations: As Alzheimer's and dementia progresses, you may find that home may not be the best place to care for your caregivee/loved one. There may come a time when you will want to consider a specialized facility that has a memory unit for the safest care of your caregivee/loved one.

9. Special Instructions Given to You by the Doctor, Nurse, or Care Team:

_____

_____

_____

_____

_____

_____

_____

_____

_____

10. Resources:
- Caregiver Resources from alzheimers.gov: http://www.alzheimers.gov/caregiver_resources.html
- Caring for Someone with alzheimers.gov: http://www.alzheimers.gov/caring.html

- About Alzheimer's Disease: Symptoms from the National Institute on Aging: http://www.nia.nih.gov/alzheimers/topics/symptoms
- Home Safety for People with Alzheimer's Disease from the National Institute on Aging: http://www.nia.nih.gov/sites/default/files/home_safety_for_people_with_alzheimers_disease.pdf
- Early-Onset Alzheimer's Disease: A Resource List from the National Institute on Aging: http://www.nia.nih.gov/alzheimers/early-onset-alzheimers-disease-resource-list?utm_source=20150302_earlyonsett&utm_medium=email&utm_campaign=ealert
- The National Institute on Aging also has the Alzheimer's Disease Education and Referral Center: http://www.nia.nih.gov/alzheimers or 1-800-438-4380
- Alzheimer's Disease from the Centers for Disease Control and Prevention: http://www.cdc.gov/aging/aginginfo/alzheimers.htm
- Alzheimer's: When To Stop Driving from the Mayo Clinic: http://www.mayoclinic.org/healthy-living/caregivers/in-depth/alzheimers/art-20044924
- Understanding Memory Loss: What To Do When You Have Trouble Remembering from the National Institute on Aging http://www.nia.nih.gov/alzheimers/publication/understanding-memory-loss/introduction?utm_source=20141222_UML&utm_medium=email&utm_campaign=ealert
- The National Institute on Aging offers the Caring for a Person with Alzheimer's Disease: Your Easy-to-Use Guide resource http://www.nia.nih.gov/alzheimers/publication/caring-person-alzheimers-disease/about-guide

- The National Institute on Aging offers "Driving Safety: Alzheimer's Caregiving Tips": https://www.nia.nih.gov/alzheimers/publication/driving-safety
- The National Institute on Aging also offers "Wandering: Alzheimer's Caregiving Tips": https://www.nia.nih.gov/alzheimers/publication/wandering

References

National Institute on Aging. About Alzheimer's Disease: Alzheimer's Basics. Retrieved from http://www.nia.nih.gov/alzheimers/topics/alzheimers-basics

AMPUTATION CARE

1. Introduction: Amputation means the loss of a limb or part of the body such as a leg, arm, hand, toe, finger, or other extremity. The cause is often from diseases that contribute to decreased circulation, such as diabetes. Severe cases of these diseases can result in amputation. According to one study, 1.6 million people were living with amputations in the United States in 2005 and that number is now estimated to be close to 2 million (Ziegler-Graham et al., 2008). It is estimated that 82% of those amputations are caused by circulatory diseases and 22% are due to trauma (Johns Hopkins Medicine, n.d.). Statistics provided by the U.S. Department of Veterans Affairs (VA) report 1,573 war-related amputations between 2001 and 2014 (VA, 2015). You will also find more amputation-specific resources listed at the end of this chapter.

You may refer to other chapters in this book such as: "Bed-bound Care (Care of the Immobilized or Bedridden Patient)," "Stroke Care (Cerebrovascular Accident)," and "Diabetes Care."

2. General Information: The loss of a limb is a very emotional and traumatic incident in a person's life. Things we take for granted, like running to answer the phone or getting up to go to the bathroom at night, are altered forever when a caregivee/loved one has to put on an artificial limb—known as a prosthesis—to even stand or walk safely. The same loss is experienced with upper extremity amputation—the loss of an arm or a hand. Sadness, anger, and frustration are common emotions that your caregivee/loved one may experience. It is important that the caregiver be understanding about the loss and allow their caregivee/loved one to do as much as possible, as safely as possible. Safety, such as avoiding falls, is especially important because it may take time for the caregivee/loved one to regain their sense of balance.

Sometimes the caregivee/loved one may complain of "phantom pain" and/or "phantom sensation" in the missing limb. Phantom pain is pain or other odd sensations experienced in the arm or leg that is no longer there. This is felt as or experienced as real pain. It may be caused by scar tissue twisting around a nerve. The pain may be described as terrible pain or, sometimes, as "weird sensations." Every person is different. Always listen to and believe your caregivee/loved one if they tell you that they have pain. Most people who have experienced an amputation will complain of pain. Sometimes phantom pain gets better over time and may no longer require treatment.

Your caregivee/loved one requires special and ongoing skin care. And this is especially true if the person uses an artificial limb. The skin on the residual limb, the part of the limb that is left after the amputation/surgery, will require special care and infection should be prevented. Learning how to use an artificial limb takes time. Physical therapy has usually been provided to help the person learn to use the new or changed prosthetic device.

3. General Goals for Care: The bottom line goals are to prevent infection and provide a safe environment. Any wound from amputation or other surgery is at risk of becoming infected because any skin opening can allow germs or dirt to enter the wound/skin and the bloodstream. If your caregivee/loved one complains of unusual or sudden soreness or pain, develops a fever, has swelling, has "shininess" or redness that doesn't go away, or has any kind of discharge (such as pus), call your doctor, nurse, or health care team right away. Infections can lead to further complications, including more surgery. As the caregiver, it is important to help your caregivee/loved one pay special attention to the skin and hygiene of the residual limb. The residual limb spends most of its time enclosed in the socket or liner of the prosthesis, and because of this it maybe more prone to skin "breakdown" and infection. Always try to prevent infection. It is *always* better to catch a problem when it is still small. It is harder for both you and your caregivee/loved one to take care of a problem when it gets big! Here are a few guidelines for taking care of the residual limb or prosthetic device.

Nutritious meals help to maintain healthy skin. The residual limb should be washed at least once a day or as directed by the prosthetist, the specialist who makes and adjusts the limb. And the area may need to be washed more often if the caregivee/loved one sweats a lot or if they are treating a rash or infection. Keep anything that comes in contact with the skin such as liners, socks, and/or the inner socket clean and dry. Having multiple liners allows the caregiver to wash one while the caregivee/loved one is wearing another. Your doctor, nurse, or other health care team member can recommend the right kind of lotion, if any, to use to keep the skin soft/protected.

The prosthetist works with the caregivee/loved one to see that their artificial limb (the *prosthetic device)* fits properly. They also work to help the person have a proper gait, or way of walking, that maintains good general muscle and bone health. The prosthetist is part of the health care team. Your caregivee/loved one will be taught how to maintain a good prosthetic fit for correct alignment and socket fit. Having the right prosthetic fit may relieve and possibly prevent pressure sores. Pressure sores can start as a red area. If a red area develops, check the prosthetic fit before the red area becomes an abrasion—a scrape or opening on the skin. Pressure from the socket/liner and the skin can cause a blister to occur. *Do not* burst a blister. Cover it with a thin, sterile dressing, check the prosthetic fit, and contact your doctor, nurse, or health care team. And of course, if your caregivee/loved one has diabetes, monitor and maintain their blood sugar levels as instructed by your doctor, nurse, or health care team. People with diabetes should examine their skin daily with a long-handled mirror or have their caregiver do so. Readers are encouraged to refer to the "Diabetes Care" chapter in this book. There is also a very damaging impact of smoking in these individuals, like all persons.

Maintain your caregivee/loved one's safety by providing well-lit areas for walking and by keeping a telephone within reach. Your caregivee/loved one may be using crutches or a walker in the home and possibly a special chair for the bath or shower for safety.

Readers are also encouraged to refer to Chapter Six: Safety in the Home: The Most Frequent Health Care Setting of Choice!

4. Personal Care Considerations: Always provide your caregivee/loved one with privacy and safety. Maintain a safe environment and always explain what you are going to do and what you are doing as you do it. Encourage your caregivee/loved one to perform their own personal care as much as possible. It is important that they be able to maintain their balance while doing this. Some people with amputations will be using crutches, a walker, or a wheelchair prior to their prosthesis being fitted. Be aware that a regular wheelchair is not balanced for an amputee and could tip over from reaching or other routine activities. Anti-tippers can be added to the wheelchair. Allow your caregivee/loved one some time to get safely comfortable. This is especially true for older persons who may take a little more time adjusting to the change and the use of crutches, a walker, or prosthetic device. Usually the prosthesis itself should not get wet (unless it is a specially designed water leg). Ask your caregivee/loved one, prosthetist, or other health care team member about the particular care and safety tips related to the prosthesis. They may provide you with a booklet on your particular prosthesis or device.

5. Safety Considerations: It is important to handle the prosthetic device gently. Prosthetic limbs are very costly. Your caregivee/loved one would be further severely handicapped in any activity if something happened to their prosthesis. And be aware that during the adjustment period to a prosthetic device, your caregivee/loved one may experience pain, discomfort, and skin problems such as sores and blisters. If this happens to your caregivee/loved one, it is time to contact the doctor, nurse, prosthetist, or other health care team member. If you or your caregivee/loved one suspects an infection, call the doctor, nurse, or health care team immediately. Prevent a small irritation from becoming a serious problem. If the doctor prescribes an antibiotic for an infection, be sure to finish all of the medication prescribed, even if the infection looks like it has gone away.

6. When to Call the Doctor, Nurse, or Care Team: These are only possible examples and NOT an inclusive list. Please remember that calling *before* a situation becomes a bigger problem is always best. It's better to catch problems when they are relatively small. It is much harder to address "big" problems.

- Caregivee/loved one develops a red or sore area that does not go away when prosthesis is off.
- Caregivee/loved one's wound feels hot, the area becomes red and/or shiny, it is swollen, and/or if there is pus or any drainage.
- Caregivee/loved one complains of a sudden increase in pain, or new severe tenderness.
- Caregivee/loved one is very emotional; perhaps they cannot stop crying or they are showing other obvious signs of distress.
- Caregivee/loved one has had a change in their bowel movements or has stopped having bowel movements for more than three days, even if they are not eating very much.
- Caregivee/loved one may be questioning their spiritual beliefs, perhaps doubting what they once believed.
- Caregivee/loved one has fallen.
- Caregivee/loved one has a sudden or high fever.
- Caregivee/loved one cannot get comfortable/find relief from pain. For example, pain wakes the caregivee/loved one up at night. Always believe whatever your caregivee/loved one tells you about their pain. Caregivee/loved ones are the expert on their pain.

- Caregivee/loved one's extremity feels cold and/or the care-givee/loved one complains of numbness or tingling in their extremity.
- The wound smells bad.
- Caregivee/loved one has swollen glands in their groin or armpits.
- Caregivee/loved one's wound has thick, brown/gray discharge or if the skin around the wound turns black.
- Any other change, complication, or concern that you or the caregivee/loved one may have. When in doubt, call!

These are examples only. Your caregivee/loved one might relay to you changes or concerns that vary from those listed here and those concerns should be addressed with your care team.

7. Comfort Considerations: Comfort for your caregivee/loved one can mean physical, mental, spiritual, or any combination of those kinds of comfort. As a caregiver, providing comfort for your caregivee/loved one sometimes means "the small things." Small things are sometimes easily overlooked. Having regular bowel movements may seem like a small thing, but it is actually a very large part of caregivee/loved one comfort. If your caregivee/loved one is on any pain medication, they can and, in many cases, do cause constipation. Sometimes your caregivee/loved one may need to take a stool softener or laxative for as long as they are on the pain medication. Unfortunately, sometimes your health care team may forget to tell you this! It is always better to prevent a problem than to correct a problem, and this is never more true than when it comes to pain medicines and constipation.

We encourage you not to be shy about asking your caregivee/ loved one about their bowel habits and call the doctor, nurse, or health care team if their bowels have not moved for three days. This is true even if they are not eating very much.

In regards to pain, changing positions or a gentle back rub and/or massage may help ease pain. Be sure to ask your caregivee/loved one's doctor or clinic before using heat or cold on your caregivee/loved one who has had amputation surgery—their skin needs very gentle treatment. Sometimes distraction, such as watching TV or a movie, reading, or playing cards is enough to ease their pain. Spending time with a beloved pet is often a wonderful therapy for those who are feeling emotionally "down" or depressed. A visit to their church or to a place that is spiritually meaningful to your caregivee/loved one, such as a drive to the ocean or other "favorite place," may comfort them spiritually. As always, your caregivee/loved one will often be the best person to guide you in what they need.

Sometimes your caregivee/loved one may ask to be left alone for awhile. Please don't take this personally! Amputation surgery disrupts a person's whole life, physically, mentally, emotionally, and, perhaps, spiritually. Their body image may be affected. Provide your caregivee/loved one time as they learn to cope with the loss of a limb and gain independence in their daily activities. The changes they experience affect those around them, including and especially the caregiver. Give your caregivee/loved one time to "regroup" if they ask for it. (And do something nice for yourself during this time!) If your caregivee/loved one doesn't recover from their need to be alone, it's time to talk to them about it and very possibly time to call the doctor, nurse, or health care team.

8. Special Considerations: The physical and mental distress caused by the loss of a limb can last for many years. Your caregivee/loved one may grieve for the loss of a limb the same as a person grieves for the loss of a loved one. Support your caregivee/loved one by being a good listener. Listen without interrupting. And no matter how comfortable a prosthetic device may be, often it's still very uncomfortable. The prosthetist or the companies that make and provide the prosthetic device are often good resources for support groups that may be of help to you both. We encourage you to consider joining a support group. Your caregivee/loved one may benefit from joining a support group for caregivee/loved ones with the same prosthetic device, or a support group of those who share the same interests including sports or other activities. And you may benefit from joining a support group for caregivers.

9. Special Instructions Given to You by the Doctor, Nurse, or Care Team:

_____

_____

_____

_____

_____

_____

_____

_____

_____

10. Resources:

- The U.S. Department of Veterans Affairs offers information on their Rehabilitation and Prosthetic Services page http://www.prosthetics.va.gov/
- The Amputee Coalition offers information about amputations and support groups http://www.amputee-coalition.org/
- MedlinePlus offers a foot amputation discharge information page including self-care guidelines http://www.nlm.nih.gov/medlineplus/ency/patientinstructions/000013.htm
- The Health Resources and Services Administration offers information about amputation through their Lower Extremity Amputation Prevention (LEAP) program's site: http://www.hrsa.gov/hansensdisease/leap/

References

Johns Hopkins Medicine. (n.d.). Amputation. Retrieved from http://www.hopkinsmedicine.org/healthlibrary/conditions/physical_medicine_and_rehabilitation/amputation_85,P01141/

U.S. Department of Veterans Affairs (VA). (2015). Prosthetics. Retrieved from http://www.research.va.gov/pubs/docs/va_factsheets/Prosthetics.pdf

Ziegler-Graham, K., MacKenzie, E. J., Ephraim, P. L., Travison, T. G., & Brookmeyer, R. (2008). Estimating the prevalence of limb loss in the United States: 2005 to 2050. *Archives of Physical Medicine and Rehabilitation*, 89(3):422–429.

ARTHRITIS CARE

1. Introduction: Arthritis is a condition of inflammation of the joints and is frequently characterized by pain and swelling. It often affects joints in the hands, knees, and hips, but it can affect many other joints. Although arthritis is primarily seen in older adults, children and young adults can also have arthritis. There are two types of arthritis: osteoarthritis, generally due to daily wear and tear to our joints which occurs over a lifetime, so it is age-related, and rheumatoid arthritis, an autoimmune inflammatory disease related to the immune system rather than age (NIH Osteoporosis and Related Bone Diseases National Resource Center, 2012). Osteoarthritis is the most common form of arthritis. Information provided by the Centers for Disease Control and Prevention (CDC) reported a survey that showed that 52.5 million U.S. adults have self-reported or doctor-diagnosed arthritis (CDC, 2013). And 22.7 million adults have limited activities due to arthritis (CDC, 2013). Juvenile arthritis (JA) and juvenile rheumatoid arthritis (JRA) are types of arthritis that impact young adults. Juvenile arthritis usually starts before the age of 16 and is a long-term or chronic illness. The CDC reported an estimated 294,000 cases of juvenile arthritis in 2007 (American College of Rheumatology, 2013).

For more information about arthritis visit: http://www.cdc.gov/arthritis. You will also find more arthritis-specific resources listed at the end of this chapter.

You may also refer to other chapters in this book such as:

"Bedbound Care (Care of the Immobilized or Bedridden Patient)" and "Older Adult Care."

2. General Information: Both osteoarthritis and rheumatoid arthritis result in pain that causes the caregivee/loved one to move slowly and to have decreased range of motion and strength. "Range of motion" is the movement that a joint can comfortably move through. For the caregiver, this means that positioning or assisting with walking must be done gently and slowly while allowing the caregivee/loved one to do as much as they can for themselves, as safely and comfortably as possible. Your patient may move more slowly in the early morning due to pain and stiffness, which may improve somewhat throughout the day.

3. General Goals for Care: Bottom line goals are that your caregivee/loved one's pain is minimized and their safety and mobility is maximized. If your caregivee/loved one takes pain medication, the medication should be taken as directed by the doctor, nurse, or health care team. It is important to take pain medication on time and to not wait too long between doses. The directions may say to take the medication "as needed;" if this is the case, the medication should be taken as soon as the patient recognizes that they are having discomfort or before doing an activity. This may prevent the pain from becoming worse. Perhaps your caregivee/loved one has been taught to use a "pain scale" and can rate their pain from a "1" (the least pain) to a "10" (the worst pain imaginable). Know your caregivee/loved one's most acceptable level of pain. For example, they may be comfortable with a level "3." Some patients may be comfortable with a level "6." The number can be very different for each person. If your caregivee/loved one's pain level is higher than usual even though they have taken their pain medication, it might be time to call the doctor, nurse, or health care team. They may want to re-evaluate your caregivee/loved one and make medication or other changes. Addressing pain earlier, rather than later, will provide the best quality of life. Never give more medication without talking to the doctor, nurse, or health care team! Always listen to and believe what your caregivee/loved one tells you about their pain. The person is the expert on the pain they are experiencing.

Your caregivee/loved one should be having regular bowel movements and this is especially important if they are on pain medication. Please call your doctor or clinic if your patient goes more than three days without a bowel movement!

Regarding safety and mobility, always help your caregivee/loved one to walk safely and remember that persons with arthritis may move very slowly. Pain and stiffness is often worse in the morning and may lessen as the day goes on. It is important that your caregivee/loved one's joints be maintained as "functional" as possible. The goal is to keep the joints comfortably and safely mobile and to preserve their ability to move. The patient's doctor, nurse, or a health care team member, such as a physical therapist, may have taught or demonstrated range of motion exercises. These exercises gently move the joint in order to keep it as supple and functional as possible. Patients with arthritis might benefit from these exercises of their fingers, hands, arms, legs, or other joints. Gentle exercise may help your caregivee/loved one maintain their ability to move safely and comfortably. Safety and comfort are always goals for any patient, regardless of their illness.

4. Personal Care Considerations: It will be important that your caregivee/loved one feels clean and comfortable, has nutritious meals, and has plenty to drink. You will want to be sure that they are urinating enough and that their urine color is not too dark. It is very important that your caregivee/loved one maintain a feeling of control over their life. Your caregivee/loved one will require patience and kindness from you, especially if they have pain or if they move very slowly because of arthritis. They should be allowed to go at their own pace and to rest between activities. Allow ample time for bathing and other personal care tasks. It may be helpful to administer pain medication, if the doctor has ordered it, a half hour to an hour before starting personal care or other exercise. As with all care, explain what you are going to do before you do it and what you are doing as you do it.

If your caregivee/loved one is especially stiff in the morning, bathing, showering, and other tasks can be accomplished later in the day. And a person with arthritis may need to conserve their energy. Let them tell you what works best for them. They may prefer short periods of activity spaced throughout the day or they may prefer having all of their personal care completed at one time, whatever works better for them. During care or between care, fingers, hands, or knees can be gently supported in their most comfortable position with small pillows or rolled up towels/facecloths. You might assist your caregivee/loved one by helping to position their hands, knees, or feet in a comfortable position. Holding a small rubber ball or a facecloth, if a rubber ball is too hard, may provide comfort and alignment for a patient with arthritis of the hand(s). If your caregivee/loved one lies on their side in bed, a pillow or rolled up towel placed under their arm may provide comfort for shoulder or arm pain. A small pillow or rolled towel placed between the knee bones and/or feet and ankle bones can provide tremendous comfort. Also, always check the patient's skin at these "boney areas" to avoid too much pressure. Change positions if you see a red area so that a wound or "pressure ulcer" does not develop. Ask your patient to guide and assist you with these measures.

Try to support your caregivee/loved one's safe independence whenever possible. For example, loosen jar tops and make sure that they can open their medicine bottles. Some pharmacies will provide easy open medication tops for patients who have arthritis in their hands. However, be mindful of children or teenagers in the house who may have access to prescribed pain medications. You may need to remind your caregivee/loved one to take their pain medication as scheduled. These gestures are thoughtful, yet allow your patient to be independent in their care.

5. Safety Considerations: The doctor, nurse, or other health care team member may suggest using bathroom aides/equipment such as grab bars, a raised toilet seat, and/or a shower chair for safety, energy conservation, and comfort. Your caregivee/loved one may be using heat or ice in addition to pain medication. Assist them to safely use these methods, being careful to use a layer of cloth between the ice or heat and the skin. The therapist can provide specific directions related to how long ice or heat should be used safely. Always check the heat temperature to make sure that your caregivee/ loved one will not be burned. If you notice that a cord on a heating pad is frayed, do not use it, replace it. Sometimes people with rheumatoid arthritis are more susceptible to infection, and for this reason it is important to maintain good infection control measures. If your caregivee/loved one develops a fever, has nausea, has changes in their urination or bowel habits, stops eating, or develops swallowing issues, it is time to call the doctor, nurse, or health care team. Sometimes, rheumatoid arthritis or treatment for rheumatoid arthritis can leave your caregivee/loved one vulnerable to mouth sores. If your caregivee/loved one complains of a mouth sore or develops white spots or a white coating on the tongue, contact the doctor, nurse, or health care team right away. Unfortunately, mouth care can be easily forgotten or may be overlooked because of discomfort or pain in the patient's hands and fingers. Because of this, your caregivee/ loved one may need assistance with their mouth care. A clean, fresh mouth helps a patient feel comfortable and it may prevent or help identify any mouth problems at an early stage.

We encourage you to read Chapter Six: Safety in the Home: The Most Frequent Health Care Setting of Choice! and Chapter Seven: Infection Control and Prevention Considerations.

6. When to Call the Doctor, Nurse, or Care Team: These are only possible examples and NOT an inclusive list. Please remember that calling *before* a situation becomes a bigger problem is always best. It's better to catch problems when they are relatively small. It is much harder to address "big" problems.

- Patient has distressful nausea or nausea that won't go away, with or without vomiting.
- Patient has stopped eating or drinking or has difficulty swallowing.
- Patient has a change in how they urinate. Perhaps they cannot urinate or they are urinating much more frequently than usual, but only producing small amounts of urine. Perhaps their urine has changed color, is very dark, and/or has a strong odor.
- Patient has had a change in their bowel movements or has stopped having bowel movements for more than three days, even if they are not eating very much.
- Patient is very emotional, perhaps they cannot stop crying or they are showing other obvious signs of distress. Perhaps they are questioning their spiritual beliefs, or doubting what they once believed.
- Patient has fallen.
- Patient has unexplained bruising or larger bruises than you would normally expect.
- Patient has a sudden or high fever.
- Patient cannot get comfortable/find relief from pain. For example, pain wakes patient up at night or pain comes on suddenly. Always believe whatever your patient tells you about their pain. Patients are the expert on their pain.
- Patient has white spots or a white coating on their tongue, or any other kind of mouth sore. This may or may not be accompanied by difficulty swallowing.
- Increased difficulty in mobility or performing tasks.
- Any other change, complication, or concern that you or the patient may have. When in doubt, call!

These are examples only. Your caregivee/loved one might relay to you changes or concerns that vary from those listed here and those concerns should be addressed with your care team.

7. Comfort Considerations: Comfort for your caregivee/loved one can mean physical, mental, spiritual, or any combination of those kinds of comfort. As a caregiver, providing comfort for your caregivee/loved one sometimes means "the small things." Small things are sometimes easily overlooked. Having regular bowel movements may seem like a small thing, but it is actually a very large part of your caregivee/loved one's comfort. If your patient is on any pain medication, they can and, in many cases, do cause constipation. Sometimes the caregivee/loved one may need to take a stool softener or laxative for as long as they are on the pain medication. Unfortunately, sometimes your health care team may forget to tell you this! It is always better to prevent a problem than to correct a problem, and this is never truer than when it comes to pain medicines and constipation. We encourage you not to be shy about asking your caregivee/loved one about their bowel habits and call the doctor, nurse, or health care team if their bowels have not moved for three days. This is true even if they are not eating very much.

In regard to discomfort or pain, changing positions, a gentle back rub, or a massage may help ease pain. A heating pad or cold/ice compress often helps with pain. Be sure to ask your patient's doctor, nurse, or health care team before using heat or cold on a patient with arthritis. And always protect your caregivee/loved one's skin by placing a cloth between their skin and the source of heat or cold. Replace any heating pad that has a frayed cord and be very careful with heating pads. Sometimes distraction, such as watching TV or a movie, reading, or playing cards is enough to ease your caregivee/loved one's discomfort. Spending time with a beloved pet is often a wonderful distraction and can help people who are feeling emotionally "down" or depressed. A visit to their place of worship or a visit from someone from their place of worship may comfort your caregivee/loved one spiritually. As always, your caregivee/loved one will often be the best person to guide you in what they need.

Sometimes your caregivee/loved one may ask to be left alone for awhile. Please don't take this personally! Having discomfort or pain and decreased mobility can really disrupt a person's whole life, and it affects those around them, including, and perhaps especially, the caregiver. Please be mindful that for a patient with arthritis, this behavior may be caused by pain that is not well controlled. We encourage you to ask your caregivee/loved one about this and address pain immediately by contacting the doctor, nurse, or health care team. Expect a quick response from a member of the care team if your caregivee/loved one is in pain. If you do not receive one, call again. No one should ever suffer in pain. If pain is not the issue, allow your caregivee/loved one time to "regroup" if they ask for it. And do something nice for yourself during this time! If your caregivee/loved one doesn't recover from their need to be alone, it's time to talk to them about it and very possibly time to call the doctor, nurse, or health care team to see if your caregivee/loved one needs to be further evaluated.

8. Special Considerations: Rheumatoid arthritis affects different people in different ways. Some patients with rheumatoid arthritis have periods of extreme pain known as "flares." Flares can be followed by periods of time when the arthritis is less painful, called "remissions." Rheumatoid arthritis is experienced physically as very painful joints, but if your caregivee/loved one has this illness they may also experience depression, anxiety, feelings of helplessness, and low self-esteem. These types of issues may impact you as caregiver. Local support groups may provide ways for both you and your loved one to maintain a sense of control during the ups and downs of this illness.

9. Special Instructions Given to You by the Doctor, Nurse, or Care Team:

_____

_____

_____

_____

_____

_____

_____

_____

_____

10. Resources:

- The Centers for Disease Control and Prevention (CDC) offers resources including basic information about arthritis: http://www.cdc.gov/arthritis
- MedlinePlus offers information about arthritis including

common types and treatment options: http://www.nlm.nih
.gov/medlineplus/ency/article/001243.htm

- The Arthritis Foundation offers information about different
types of arthritis as well as tips for eating well and staying
active on their website: http://www.arthritis.org/

- The Arthritis Foundation also offers a resource specifically
for caregivers: http://www.arthritistoday.org/what-you-can-
do/everyday-solutions/caregiving/

- The National Institute of Arthritis and Musculoskeletal
and Skin Diseases offers an information page about rheumatoid arthritis in particular: http://www.niams.nih.gov/
health_info/rheumatic_disease/rheumatoid_arthritis_ff.asp

References

American College of Rheumatology (2013). Prevalence Statistics. Retrieved
from http://www.rheumatology.org/Research/Prevalence_Statistics/

Centers for Disease Control (CDC). (2013). Prevalence of Doctor-
Diagnosed Arthritis and Arthritis-Attributable Activity Limitation—
United States, 2010–2012. Retrived from http://www.cdc.gov/mmwr/
preview/mmwrhtml/mm6244a1.htm

NIH Osteoporosis and Related Bone Diseases National Resource Center.
(2012). Osteoporosis and Arthritis: Two Common but Different Conditions. Retrieved from http://www.niams.nih.gov/health_info/bone/
Osteoporosis/Conditions_Behaviors/osteoporosis_arthritis.asp

BEDBOUND CARE
(CARE OF THE IMMOBILIZED OR BEDRIDDEN PATIENT)

1. Introduction: Persons who are immobilized and confined to bed are considered "bedbound." Causes of immobility vary and illness and injury can cause someone to temporarily or permanently be bedbound. Your caregivee/loved one may be confined to a bed or they may have the ability to transfer with assistance between the bed and a chair, but, in general, they do not have the ability to reposition themselves or to move about independently. Those who are bedbound have special needs because immobility causes changes and problems to all of the different body "systems." These systems include the skin, the muscles and bones, the cardiac or heart system, the respiratory or breathing system, the immune system (which protects people from infection), the urinary system and the food processing system (which includes both eating and eliminating food). And because these systems are all "interwoven" in the body, one system almost always affects another.

Due to immobility, many of the bedbound person's body systems are "compromised" or impacted in some other negative way. A caregivee/loved one who is bedbound may have a poor appetite. Depression can add to the poor appetite noted in many bedbound caregivee/loved ones. This could cause poor nutrition and this may affect wound healing should the person develop a wound or pressure ulcer. If the caregivee/loved one does not get exercise, their muscles and bones are affected and they may experience muscle wasting. This means their muscles may become thin and weak. The bedbound person's circulation (the heart system, which is needed for general good health) may function poorly because of a lack of exercise. This lack of exercise can contribute to other problems, including blood clots. Lying flat in a bed for a long time can negatively affect the lungs and cause a lung or other infection, such as pneumonia. Constipation and depression are other complications of immobility.

As the caregiver of a bedbound person, you may need to learn to assess and protect your caregivee/loved one's skin and their ability to eat nutritious meals safely. You may need to become mindful of other aspects of their care as well, such as mobility issues, blood circulation issues, breathing issues, and incontinence.

You may also refer to other chapters in this book such as: "Alzheimer's Disease and Dementia Care," "Amputation Care," "Arthritis Care," "Cancer Care," "Cardiac Care," "Stroke Care (Cerebrovascular Accident)," "Chronic Obstructive Pulmonary Disease (COPD) Care," "End-of-Life Care," "Older Adult Care," and "Urinary and Incontinence Care."

2. General Information: The biggest risk to those who are bedbound are what were historically called "bedsores," also called "pressure ulcers." They are caused by constant pressure on one area of the body. Unrelieved pressure on skin areas causes damage to the underlying tissue, the tissue that cannot be seen, below the level of the skin. These sores often occur over boney areas, or prominences, such as at the base of the spine or on the shoulder blades, heels, elbows, on the sides of the knees, hips, or at the back of the head. They can occur anywhere on the skin where there is constant, unrelieved pressure. In many cases, pressure sores can be prevented. It is always better to prevent a problem than to address a problem, and this is especially true with pressure sores. Pressure sores can be uncomfortable and painful and can become infected. If your caregivee/loved one is incontinent, the wound may become soiled and this could lead to a very serious infection. In addition, when the ability to feel pressure/pain is diminished, the risk for pressure ulcers or complicated wound healing is increased.

These wounds, if they occur, can also be very hard to heal. Proper nutrition and frequent position changes can contribute to your caregivee/loved one having healthy, intact skin. If you see an area of redness on your caregivee/loved one's skin, assist them in changing positions so that pressure is relieved from that area. If the red area does not go away, it is important to contact the doctor, nurse, or health care team right away. The person's doctor, nurse, or health care team may recommend deep breathing or coughing exercises to help prevent lung infections and range of motion exercises to help the person's muscles, bones, and circulatory systems.

For more information about pressure sores, the University of Washington offers a pamphlet called "Taking Care of Pressure Sores": http://sci.washington.edu/info/pamphlets/takecare_pressuresores.pdf. You will find more care-of-the-bedbound-caregivee/loved one-specific resources listed at the end of this chapter.

3. General Goals for Care: Bottom line goal is twofold and includes both you and your caregivee/loved one. Both goals are equally important!

a. The goal for your caregivee/loved one is that they are safe and comfortable, have nutritious meals, have plenty to drink, experience minimal discomfort or pain, and have minimal anxiety. And they need to be kept free from infections. Even people who are bedbound need periods of rest and some form of exercise, such as gentle range of motion exercises, each day. Ask your doctor or health care provider about this. Consistency in daily activities provides a sense of safety and comfort. Everyone needs to feel that they have a sense of control of their lives. Give them this as much as possible. They should be allowed to go at their own pace. If they are able, encourage them to choose their meals, feed themselves, and perform as much of their own personal care tasks as possible.

It is important that your caregivee/loved one's joints and muscles be maintained as "functional" as possible. The goal is to keep the bones, joints, and muscles moving safely, to preserve their ongoing ability to move. The person's doctor, nurse, or a health care team member, such as a physical therapist, may have taught or demonstrated range of motion exercises for your caregivee/loved one. These exercises gently move the limbs in order to keep the joints and muscles as supple and functional as possible. People who are bedbound may benefit from these exercises of their fingers, hands, arms, legs, or other joints. Gentle exercise may help your caregivee/loved one prevent muscle wasting and maintain their ability to move safely and comfortably. And it is good to remember that they may be experiencing pain and stiffness due to immobility. If your caregivee/loved one is experiencing pain, be sure to contact the doctor, nurse, or health care team right away. No caregivee/loved one should be in pain and immobility can cause pain in the bedbound caregivee/loved one. Always believe what your caregivee/loved one tells you about pain and remember that they are the experts about their pain.

For more pain management information, please see the section on "Arthritis Care" in this book. If your caregivee/loved one is unable to speak, watch for signs of pain that are "non-verbal." Moaning, grimacing, crying out when being moved, and/or a furrowed brow are all signs of pain. Always address your caregivee/loved one's pain immediately. It is often a good idea to give pain medication a half hour to an hour before they receive care that requires movement. This is called "pre-medication" and it shows caring and kindness on your part. Ask your caregivee/loved one's doctor, nurse, or health care team about pre-medicating for pain. Comfort is always a goal for any caregivee/loved one, regardless of their illness.

You will want to always be sure that your caregivee/loved one is urinating enough and that their urine color is light in color. Your caregivee/loved one should be having regular bowel movements and this is especially important if they are on pain medication. People taking pain medications usually need a stool softener or laxative because most pain medications cause constipation. They may need to take it daily while on pain medication. Please call the doctor or clinic if your caregivee/loved one goes more than three days without a bowel movement! Later in this chapter you will find more specific information about ways to help people who are bedbound to be as comfortable as possible.

Your caregivee/loved one may be completely bedbound or they may be bed-to-chairbound—still able to sit in a chair. If they can sit in a chair, always help them to transfer to the chair safely and slowly. The doctor, nurse, or health care team may make recommendations about equipment to use in the home, such as a "gait belt" and/or "slide board" to help your caregivee/loved one to safely transfer from a bed to a chair and back. These could also include beds, bed rails, support stockings, or other equipment. A shower chair can also benefit by providing safety, comfort, and energy conservation. A urinal and/or a bedpan may be helpful. As the caregiver, you should be instructed on the proper use of any equipment that is recommended. Often a physical therapist is part of the health care team and they may demonstrate the proper use of equipment, and good "body mechanic" techniques, for you to keep both you and your caregivee/loved one safe during position changes and transfers.

Your caregivee/loved one's skin should be assessed every day and this will become a part of their everyday care during bath or personal care activities time. It is a good idea to "get in the habit" of always observing their skin as you provide any care throughout the day. Having a consistent caregiver benefits the caregivee/loved one by having someone who will notice any new red areas or other changes in the skin. Every caregiver involved with your caregivee/loved one should be taught to be observant of possible skin problems and to address them and report these right away. The person must be repositioned carefully and gently. Care should be taken to minimize the force and friction applied to the skin during position changes. Be cautious not to "shear" the person's skin. "Shearing" mean causing an abrasion or cut on the skin and is caused by pulling or dragging sheets out from under them. Your caregivee/loved one's bed linens should be dry and clean. Your caregivee/loved one should lie on bed linens that are smooth and wrinkle-free. The doctor, nurse, or health care team can show you techniques to safely turn and reposition your caregivee/loved one, how to help a person onto a bedpan, and how to make a bed with a person in it.

Infection control is important for everyone and, for a caregivee/loved one who is immobile, this is especially true. Their immune system may not be strong enough to fight infections. For your caregivee/loved one, good nutrition, plenty to drink, gentle exercises for range of motion or flexibility, and intact skin may help to prevent infection. As always, with any personal care, wash your hands, wash your hands, wash your hands!

b. It is very important that you, as caregiver, maintain a sense of control over your life. The person who is bedbound can become very dependent upon one person (you!) for care. This is because they depend upon consistency in order to feel safe. As caregiver, you are at risk of becoming physically, and mentally, fatigued. If your caregivee/loved one is experiencing depression, this can affect you as well. As the caregiver, you may benefit from the support resources listed at the end of this chapter. We strongly encourage you to seek local resources, perhaps at churches or community centers near you, for support groups or meetings. Patience and kindness from you toward your caregivee/loved one and toward yourself is in order here. You may need to find a way to take time out from the repetition of caring for the caregivee/loved one who is bedbound. The doctor, nurse, or health care team may be able to provide you with information about caregivers in your local community. A social worker may be part of your health care team and may be able to provide you with information about local resources. Do not try to go it alone. Caring for a bedbound person is a tremendous amount of work. If at all possible, enlist the help of others, such as family members or friends who offer to help.

4. Personal Care Considerations: Your caregivee/loved one may have an indwelling urinary catheter and may be incontinent of their bowels. Meticulous skin care is important in maintaining skin that is free of reddened areas that can become open wounds known as pressure sores. If your caregivee/loved one is incontinent, cleanse their skin with mild soap and water, rinse, if possible, and gently pat—do not rub—the skin dry. Address soiling immediately if possible. Urine and stool, when left on the skin, quickly contribute to skin breakdown. The doctor, nurse, or health care team may recommend the use of "baby wipes" or other disposable products, and they may recommend products that do not contain alcohol. When moisture cannot be controlled, such as with urinary incontinence, use under-pads or adult incontinence briefs that are absorbent and present a quick-drying surface to the skin. Your doctor, nurse, or health care team may direct you to use a special skin lotion that protects the skin. Contact them before using any product on your caregivee/loved one's skin. You may be directed to use a special mattress, such as an alternating pressure mattress or a dense foam mattress, to prevent pressure areas/skin break down. This may also provide extra comfort to the caregivee/loved one. These special mattresses or foam pads are also available for wheelchairs and may be recommended if your caregivee/loved one sits a lot. Oftentimes, insurance will cover part of the costs of these items.

Your caregivee/loved one who is bedbound may or may not be able to help with part of their care. They may be able to help with repositioning themselves in bed for example. They may be able to help with transferring from the bed to the chair and back again. Doing this may help them to preserve a feeling of dignity and independence. They may need to conserve their energy in order to help with these tasks. Let them tell you what works best for them. They may prefer short periods of activity spaced throughout the day or perhaps having all of their personal care completed at one time works better for them. Always remember that safety is key. Protect your caregivee/loved one from falls at all times.

If your caregivee/loved one is unable to assist in their personal care, they may benefit, during care and/or between care, by having their fingers, hands, or knees gently supported with small pillows or rolled up towels/facecloths. You might assist them by helping place their hands, knees, or feet in a comfortable position. Holding a small rubber ball/facecloth may provide comfort and alignment in the hands of a caregivee/loved one who is immobile. If your caregivee/loved one lies on their side, a pillow or rolled up towel placed under their arm may provide comfort for shoulder or arm pain. And a small pillow or rolled towel placed between the knee bones and/or feet and ankle bones can provide tremendous comfort. Also, always check your caregivee/loved one's skin at these "boney areas" and avoid bone to bone contact. Change their position if you see a red area so that a wound or "pressure sore" does not develop! Ask your caregivee/loved one to tell you what feels right for them. And always, with all care, explain to them what you are going to do and what you are doing as you do it.

Bedbound people are also at risk for what is called "foot drop." This is a condition that causes the person to experience difficulty in lifting up the foot. It is best to prevent foot drop. Ask the doctor, nurse, or health care team about special positioning, equipment, or other supportive devices sometimes called a "foot board" or "foot cradle" to prevent this problem. Wearing tennis shoes may help some people and this is something to ask the doctor, nurse, or health care team about.

Your caregivee/loved one's bed bath is an important part of total care. It maintains hygiene and helps keep them clean and comfortable. Be aware of the temperature of the water as your caregivee/loved one may be very sensitive to hot and cold. Avoid hot water! Fall safety is a big concern when bathing a caregivee/loved one who is bedbound. Allow and encourage them to participate in their bath routine as much as possible. They may be able to wash their face and neck, for example, or to perform their own mouth care. As caregiver, your task may be to "set them up" with the items they need. Unfortunately, mouth care can be easily forgotten or overlooked, but it is an important part of daily hygiene because the bedbound caregivee/loved one may be vulnerable to mouth and throat infections. A clean, fresh mouth adds to the caregivee/loved one's quality of life. It helps them to taste food and aids in digestion. Daily mouth care may prevent or help identify any mouth problems at an early stage. If your caregivee/loved one complains of a sore mouth or develops white spots or a white coating on the tongue, contact the doctor, nurse, or health care team right away.

Always protect your caregivee/loved one's dignity and privacy. During bathing, keep them covered, only expose the body part that is actually being bathed. And keep your caregivee/loved one warm during bath time. You can use an extra bath or beach towel for warmth and privacy. Use moisturizer after bathing if advised by the doctor, nurse, or health care team. This is a good way to show caring through gentle touch. The bed bath is a perfect time to assess your caregivee/loved one's skin. And always protect their skin by never using hot water. We encourage you to ask your doctor, nurse, or other health care team members to teach you and your caregivee/loved one about proper positioning, transferring, and turning techniques. And remember that good "body mechanics" may protect you and the caregivee/loved one from injury.

5. Safety Considerations: People who are bedbound may be very susceptible to infection. For this reason, it is important to maintain good infection control measures. Always wash your hands before touching your caregivee/loved one, and, of course, after providing any personal care. Wearing gloves is another infection control consideration. Always wash your hands after removing gloves also. If your caregivee/loved one develops a fever, has nausea, has changes in their urination or bowel habits, has sudden severe pain, stops eating, or develops swallowing issues, it is time to call the doctor, nurse, or health care team. If your caregivee/loved one starts to behave differently from how they usually behave or if they show signs of confusion or a personality change, this may be a sign of a urinary tract infection, especially in older adults. Call the doctor, nurse, or health care team right away if this happens. If the doctor prescribes medication for an infection, it is important to give it as directed. Always have your caregivee/loved one finish antibiotic medications even if they start to feel better. If you are unsure if the medication prescribed is an antibiotic, call the doctor, nurse, or health care team member and/or ask the pharmacist.

We encourage you to read Chapter Six: Safety in the Home: The Most Frequent Health Care Setting of Choice! and Chapter Seven: Infection Control and Prevention Considerations.

6. When to Call the Doctor, Nurse, or Care Team: These are only possible examples and NOT an inclusive list. Please remember that calling *before* a situation becomes a bigger problem is always best. It's better to catch problems when they are relatively small. It is much harder to address "big" problems.

- Caregivee/loved one has an area of redness on their skin that does not go away shortly after repositioning them.
- Caregivee/loved one has distressful nausea or nausea that won't go away, with or without vomiting.
- Caregivee/loved one has stopped eating or drinking or has difficulty swallowing.
- Caregivee/loved one has a change in how they urinate. Perhaps they cannot urinate or they are urinating much more frequently than usual, but only producing small amounts of urine. Perhaps their urine has changed color, is very dark and/or has a strong odor.
- Caregivee/loved one has had a change in their bowel movements or has stopped having bowel movements for more than three days, even if they are not eating very much.
- Caregivee/loved one has fallen.
- Caregivee/loved one experiences sudden chest pain.
- Caregivee/loved one experiences throbbing pain in an extremity (arm, hand, leg, foot).
- Caregivee/loved one has a cold extremity. This could include no pulse in an extremity or redness, shininess, or swelling above a cold limb.
- Caregivee/loved one has unexplained bruising, or larger bruises than you would normally expect.

- Caregivee/loved one has facial drooping on one side of their face.
- Caregivee/loved one experiences a loss of feeling or a loss of movement in one of their limbs.
- Caregivee/loved one has a sudden or high fever.
- Caregivee/loved one shows a personality change and/or has an increase in confusion.
- Caregivee/loved one cannot get comfortable/find relief from pain. For example, pain wakes caregivee/loved one up at night, or pain comes on suddenly. Always believe whatever your caregivee/loved one tells you about their pain. Caregivee/loved ones are the expert on their pain.
- Caregivee/loved one has white spots or a white coating on their tongue, or any other kind of mouth sore. This may or may not be accompanied by difficulty swallowing.
- Caregivee/loved one is very emotional, perhaps they cannot stop crying or they are showing other obvious signs of distress.
- Caregivee/loved one is questioning their spiritual beliefs, perhaps doubting what they once believed.
- Any other change, complication, or concern that you or the caregivee/loved one may have. When in doubt, call!

These are examples only. Your caregivee/loved one might relay to you changes or concerns that vary from those listed here and those concerns should be addressed with your care team.

7. Comfort Considerations: Comfort for your caregivee/loved one can mean physical, mental, spiritual, or any combination of those kinds of comfort. As a caregiver, providing comfort sometimes means "the small things." Small things are sometimes easily overlooked. Having regular bowel movements may seem like a small thing, but it is actually a very large part of your caregivee/loved one's comfort.

If your caregivee/loved one is on any pain medication, they can and, in many cases, do cause constipation. Sometimes they may need to take a stool softener or laxative for as long as they are on the pain medication. Unfortunately, sometimes your health care team may forget to tell you this! It is always better to prevent a problem than to correct a problem, and this is never more true than when it comes to pain medicines and constipation. We encourage you not to be shy about talking with your caregivee/loved one about their bowel habits and call the doctor, nurse or health care team if their bowels have not moved for three days. This is true even if they are not eating very much.

In regard to discomfort or pain, changing positions, a gentle back rub or massage may help ease pain. A heating pad, or cold/ice compress often helps with pain. Be sure to ask your caregivee/loved one's doctor, nurse, or health care team before using heat or cold on a caregivee/loved one who is bedbound. And always protect your caregivees/loved one's skin by placing a cloth between their skin and the source of heat or cold. Replace any heating pad that has a frayed cord and be very careful with heating pads. People who are bedbound have very fragile skin. Sometimes, distraction, such as watching TV or a movie, reading, or playing cards will ease a caregivee/loved one's discomfort. Spending time with a beloved pet is often a wonderful distraction and can help people who are feeling emotionally "down" or depressed. A visit from someone from their church or place of worship may comfort your caregivee/loved one spiritually. As always, your caregivee/loved one will often be the best person to guide you, by telling you what they need.

8. Special Considerations: If/as your caregivee/loved one's needs progress, you may find that home may not be the best place to provide care. There may come a time when you will want to consider a specialized facility for the safest care of your caregivee/loved one. Start this conversation with your caregivee/loved one, primary care provider, nurse practitioner, or other health care team member. They will usually have information about local health care resources and facilities or can refer you to those who have this information.

9. Special Instructions Given to You by the Doctor, Nurse, or Care Team:

_____

_____

_____

_____

_____

_____

_____

_____

10. Resources:

- MedlinePlus offers an information page about pressure sores: http://www.nlm.nih.gov/medlineplus/pressuresores .html

- MedlinePlus also offers information about preventing pressure ulcers and what signs to watch out for: https://medlineplus.gov/ency/patientinstructions/000147.htm
- Medline Plus also has a page of information on correctly moving a caregivee/loved one in bed to avoid hurting either yourself or the caregivee/loved one: https://medlineplus.gov/ency/patientinstructions/000429.htm
- The New Jersey Hospital Association Institute of Quality and Patient Safety have a resource available called the "Pressure Ulcer Prevention Change Package": http://www.njha.com/media/40907/put_changepackage.pdf

CANCER CARE

1. Introduction: The National Cancer Institute (NCI) estimates that in 2016, an estimated 1,685,210 new cases of cancer will be diagnosed in the United States and 595,690 will die from the disease. The number of people living beyond a cancer diagnosis reached nearly 14.5 million in 2014 and is expected to rise to almost 19 million by 2024. (NCI, n.d.). For more Cancer specific information and statistics, visit the NCI website at: http://www.cancer.gov/. You will also find more Cancer-specific resources listed at the end of this chapter.

Cancers vary widely and include blood disorders, such as leukemia, as well as solid tumors, such as lung or stomach "tumors," sometimes referred to as "masses" or "growths." Metastases are cancer sites that have moved from the original cancer sites. Cancer affects people of all ages, from the very young to the very old.

You may also refer to other chapters in this book such as: "Bedbound Care (Care of the Immobilized or Bedridden Patient)," "Chronic Obstructive Pulmonary Disease (COPD) Care," "End-of-Life Care," and "Urinary and Incontinence Care."

2. General Information: Caring for a person diagnosed with cancer may feel overwhelming, but the statistics above show that you are not alone! And people who have experienced cancer tend to have had a long history of interactions with their professional health care team. If this describes your caregivee/ loved one, he/she may well be the "expert" on their particular kind of cancer and the care they need. In many cases, the person has received written information from their doctors and nurses that tells them how to care for their specific needs. It is very important to follow these instructions. If you have questions about these written instructions, for example, "How long do we keep the bandage on?" or "Can he shower with it?" it is recommended that you call the doctor's office or clinic where your caregivee/loved one had their treatment to ask for specific guidance. In addition, because of the complex variations of kinds of cancer and cancer treatments, it is always recommended that any new changes, symptoms, or concerns that the person experiences be addressed by calling the cancer clinic where your caregivee/loved one was treated.

People who have been diagnosed with cancer often feel that they have lost control of their lives. It is important to allow them to direct their care as much as possible so they maintain a sense of control. Cancer affects the immediate family, the extended family, and the friends of the person. Cancer also affects the caregivers, have no doubt! It is for this reason that we must be sensitive not only to the needs of the person but also to the self-care of you, the caregiver, as well. Please refer to Chapter Eight of this book "Self-Care of the Caregiver (Taking Care of Yourself!)" for more information.

3. General Goals for Care: The bottom line goals are that your caregivee/loved one feels clean and comfortable, has nutritious meals, has plenty to drink, and has minimal discomfort, pain, and/or anxiety. It is very important that they maintain a feeling of control over their life. Your caregivee/loved one will likely require some emotional support as well, which simply means patience and kindness (from you). They may need you to listen to their story of their illness, perhaps many times, without interruption. Often, their self-image has suffered, especially if their body has changed or if they have suffered hair loss. This is true for both men and women. They especially need plenty of rest because of the way their treatment affects their bodies. They should be allowed to go at their own pace and to rest between activities. You will want to always be sure that your caregivee/loved one is urinating enough and that their urine color is not too dark in color. They should be having regular bowel movements, and this is especially important if they are on pain medication. Please call your caregivee/loved one's doctor or clinic if they go more than three days without a bowel movement! Comfort is always a goal for any person, regardless of their illness. Below you will find a section of this chapter that provides information about ways to help your caregivee/loved one be comfortable.

4. Personal Care Considerations: Those who have been diagnosed with cancer may have experienced surgery, chemotherapy, radiation, or a combination of these treatments. The resources at the end of this chapter will guide you in helping to manage many of the symptoms your caregivee/loved one may be experiencing.

    Caregivee/loved ones who have had CHEMOTHERAPY: May feel very tired; have lost their hair; bruise easily; and be nauseated, with or without vomiting. The sight or smell of food or specific foods may also make some people feel sick so keep this in mind when cooking for yourself and your family. They may also have pain, discomfort, or other symptoms.

    Caregivee/loved ones who have had RADIATION: May feel

very weak/tired. They may also have diarrhea. They may have redness of their skin, similar to sunburn. It's best to *only* apply lotions or powders to the skin that have been recommended by the doctors, nurses, or clinic where the caregivee/loved one received their treatment.

Cancer, and some treatments for cancer, makes the person more vulnerable to catching colds or influenza (flu). They may need to wear a mask when they go out in public. And if you, the caregiver, have a cold or flu, if you are coughing or sneezing or have a fever, it is recommended that you wear a mask to protect your caregivee/loved one while you are providing them with care. It may be helpful to refer to Chapter Seven: Infection Control and Prevention Considerations for more information. Cancer caregivee/loved ones do not have a strong ability to fight infections, so prevention is key.

Caregivee/loved ones who have had SURGERY: May feel very weak/tired. They may also have pain at the incision site of the surgery. The caregiver should ask the doctor and/or surgery center for specific care after surgery.

5. Safety Considerations: A person with cancer may also have bones that break more easily than usual, similar to the bones of older people. Because of this, it is important to prevent falls and to try to create a safe environment. In fall situations where you might only suffer a sore arm with a black and blue mark, a person with cancer may have a broken arm. Because those with cancer are more at risk for breaking a bone, always remember "safety first" when helping your caregivee/loved one with walking or changing from one position to another. As part of your own self-care, be mindful of your own body mechanics so that you stay healthy too! Any changes associated with your caregivee/loved one's mobility should be reported to the doctor or clinic right away. And any large bruises or bruises that seem to appear without reason should be reported to the doctor or clinic as well. Readers are encouraged to refer to Chapter Six of this book: "Safety in the Home."

6. When to Call the Doctor, Nurse, or Care Team: These are only possible examples and NOT an inclusive list. Please remember that calling *before* a situation becomes a bigger problem is always best. It's better to catch problems when they are relatively small. It is much harder to address "big" problems.

- Caregivee/loved one is very emotional, perhaps they cannot stop crying or they are showing other obvious signs of distress.
- Caregivee/loved one has distressful nausea or nausea that won't go away, with or without vomiting.
- Caregivee/loved one has stopped eating or drinking or has difficulty swallowing.
- Caregivee/loved one has a change in how they urinate. Perhaps they cannot urinate or they are urinating much more frequently than usual, but only producing small amounts of urine. Perhaps their urine has changed color, is very dark, and/or has a strong odor.
- Caregivee/loved one has had a change in their bowel movements or has stopped having bowel movements for more than three days, even if they are not eating very much.
- Caregivee/loved one may be questioning their spiritual beliefs, perhaps doubting what they once believed.
- Caregivee/loved one has fallen.

- Caregivee/loved one has unexplained bruising or larger bruises than you would normally expect.
- Caregivee/loved one has a sudden or high fever.
- Caregivee/loved one cannot get comfortable/find relief from pain. For example, pain wakes caregivee/loved one up at night or pain comes on suddenly. Always believe whatever your caregivee/loved one tells you about their pain. Caregivee/loved ones are the expert on their pain.
- Caregivee/loved one has white spots or a white coating on their tongue or any other kind of mouth sore. This may or may not be accompanied by difficulty swallowing.
- Increase in arm or leg edema.
- Any other change, complication, or concern that you or the caregivee/loved one may have. When in doubt, call!

These are examples only. Your caregivee/loved one might relay to you changes or concerns that vary from those listed here and those concerns should be addressed with your care team.

7. Comfort Considerations: Comfort for your caregivee/loved one can mean physical, mental, spiritual, or any combination of those kinds of comfort. As a caregiver, providing comfort for your caregivee/loved one sometimes means "the small things." Small things are sometimes easily overlooked. Having regular bowel movements may seem like a small thing, but it is actually a very large part of comfort. If your caregivee/loved one is on any pain medication, they can and, in many cases, do cause constipation. Sometimes the caregivee/loved one may need to take a stool softener or laxative for as long as they are on the pain medication.

Unfortunately, sometimes your health care team may forget to tell you this! It is always better to prevent a problem than to correct a problem, and this is never more true than when it comes to pain medicines and constipation. We encourage you not to be shy about asking your caregivee/loved one about their bowel habits and call the doctor or clinic if their bowels have not moved for three days. This is true even if they are not eating very much.

In regards to pain, changing positions or a gentle back rub/massage may help ease pain. A heating pad or cold/ice compress can often help with pain. Be sure to ask your caregivee/loved one's doctor or clinic before using heat or cold on a caregivee/loved one who has had radiation treatment—their skin needs very gentle treatment. Sometimes distraction, such as watching TV or a movie, reading, or playing cards is enough to ease a caregivee/loved one's pain. Spending time with a beloved pet is often a wonderful therapy for those who are feeling emotionally "down" or depressed. A visit to their church or to a place that is spiritually meaningful to your caregivee/loved one, such as a drive to the ocean, may comfort them spiritually. As always, your caregivee/loved one will often be the best person to guide you in what they need.

Sometimes your caregivee/loved one may ask to be left alone for a while. Please don't take this personally! Having cancer really disrupts a person's whole life, and, again, it affects those around them, including, and especially, the caregiver. Give your caregivee/loved one time to "regroup" if they ask for it. (And do something nice for yourself during this time!) If your caregivee/loved one doesn't recover from their need to be alone after a day or two, it's time to talk to them about it and very possibly time to call the doctor or clinic.

A clean fresh mouth helps a person feel comfortable and may head off problems of the mouth at an early stage. Sometimes, cancer or cancer treatment causes mouth sores or a white coating on the tongue and, as stated previously, this is something you want to contact the doctor or clinic about.

8. Special Considerations: Sometimes, as a person approaches the end of life, the caregivee/loved one, the doctor, and the caregiver may wish to consider either palliative care or hospice care. For more information and resources related to these types of care, please refer to the chapter entitled "End-of-Life, Palliative, and Hospice Care."

9. Special Instructions Given to You by the Doctor, Nurse, or Care Team:

_____

_____

_____

_____

_____

_____

_____

_____

_____

10. Resources:

- Coping with Cancer from the National Cancer Institute: http://www.cancer.gov/cancertopics/coping
- Organizations and Resources from the National Cancer Institute: http://www.cancer.gov/cancertopics/aya/resources

- Cancer Treatment from the National Cancer Institute: http://www.cancer.gov/cancertopics/treatment
- Complementary and Alternative Resources from the National Cancer Institute: http://www.cancer.gov/cancertopics/cam
- Caring for the Caregiver from the National Cancer Institute: http://www.cancer.gov/publications/patient-education/caring-for-the-caregiver
- Caregiving Resources from the Centers for Disease Control and Prevention: http://www.cdc.gov/cancer/survivorship/caregivers/resources.htm
- Breast Cancer Awareness from the Centers for Disease Control and Prevention: http://www.cdc.gov/cancer/dcpc/resources/features/BreastCancerAwareness/
- The Health Affairs Blog featured a story from Amy Berman about her perspective on treatment and (potential) overtreatment for cancer: http://healthaffairs.org/blog/2014/05/22/narrative-matters-the-next-chapter-amy-berman-reflects-on-living-life-in-my-own-way/
- There is also a talk from Amy Berman on the NIH's website: http://videocast.nih.gov/summary.asp?Live=11519&bhcp=1
- Support for People with Oral and Head and Neck Cancer is a support group for caregivee/loved ones and families suffering from this cancer that also has local chapters throughout the United States: https://www.spohnc.org

Reference

National Cancer Institute (NCI). (n.d.). SEER Stat Fact Sheets: All Cancer Sites. Retrieved from http://seer.cancer.gov/statfacts/html/all.html

CARDIAC CARE

1. Introduction: Cardiac caregivee/loved ones are people with heart problems. These problems include: changes in the blood vessels that supply the heart tissue; a weakening of the heart's ability to pump; or an irregular heartbeat, called an arrhythmia (ah-rith-me-ah). You may hear cardiac or heart problems referred to as "coronary" disease. As a caregiver, you may be providing care to a caregivee/loved one after a heart attack, following heart surgery, or experiencing an illness known as "heart failure." You may be caring for someone with a heart arrhythmia. Because the range of heart diseases are complex and wide ranging, your caregivee/loved one's doctor will provide you with more specific information about the type of heart ailment that your caregivee/loved one has. It might be helpful to have a basic understanding of how the heart works and the caregivee/loved one's doctor may have shown you a model of a human heart.

The heart is a muscle about the size of a fist. It is located in the center of the chest and it is the body's "pump," pumping oxygen rich blood, which it picks up from the nearby lungs, and delivering it throughout the body. The heart pumps blood from the chest to both the top of the head and to the feet and then the blood returns to the heart (the "circulation"). All muscles need a good blood/oxygen supply to work properly, the heart included. Without oxygen, muscles can become weak or even damaged. For more information on the anatomy and physiology of the heart, visit the National

Heart, Lung, and Blood Institute's "Explore How the Heart Works" page: http://www.nhlbi.nih.gov/health/health-topics/topics/hhw.

Heart disease is the leading cause of death in the United States for both men and women (Centers for Disease Control and Prevention [CDC], 2015). The CDC reports that more than 600,000 people die in the U.S. every year and 1 in 4 deaths are caused by heart disease (CDC, 2015). Each year, about 735,000 people in the U.S. have a heart attack (CDC, 2015). For more than half of those people, 525,000, it is their first heart attack; the remaining 210,000 people have already experienced a heart attack (CDC, 2015). For more information about heart disease visit: http://www.cdc.gov/heart disease. You will find more cardiac-specific resources listed at the end of this chapter.

The most common heart disease is called "coronary artery disease" (CAD) and it is the number one cause of heart attacks (National Heart, Lung, and Blood Institute, 2013). CAD is caused by atherosclerosis (ath-er-oh-scler-osis), which is a build-up of waxy-like, fatty deposits, or plaque, inside the blood vessels that supply blood to all parts of the body, including the heart (National Heart, Lung, and Blood Institute, 2013). Atherosclerosis, or "hardening of the arteries," can happen anywhere in the body and when it occurs, blood flow is restricted because the blood vessels become too narrow, stiffened, or even clogged. When this happens to the blood vessels that supply the heart muscle, known as the coronary arteries, it can lead to a heart attack. Many people survive heart attacks and go on to live full and healthy lives. Atherosclerosis is not a normal part of aging. It can be caused by risk factors which include high blood pressure, high cholesterol, diabetes, obesity, a lack of physical exercise or activity, and/or smoking.

Another common form of heart disease is called "heart failure," also known as "congestive heart failure" (CHF). As a caregiver, you may be caring for someone who has this diagnosis. Heart failure or CHF is a frightening name, but it does not mean that the heart has "failed" or has stopped beating. It means that the heart is not pumping effectively, which can cause fluid to back up in both the lungs and the legs. Heart failure (HF) is one of the most common reasons for hospitalizations of persons age 65 and older (CDC, 2012).

Other kinds of heart problems can occur when the heart has an irregular heartbeat, called an arrhythmia. An arrhythmia is when a heart beats too fast, too slow, or with an irregular rhythm. The most common type of heart arrhythmia is called Atrial Fibrillation (A-tree-al fib-rill-a-shun), commonly referred to as "A-Fib." A-fib or AF is caused when the two upper chambers of the heart contract rapidly and irregularly. Under normal circumstances, an electrical system within the heart causes the heart to pump at a regular rate and rhythm. A disruption of this electrical system can lead to AF if the rate and rhythm becomes disorganized and rapid. The heart has four chambers. When the two upper chambers are pumping rapidly and irregularly (fibrillating), the two lower chambers of the heart do not receive enough blood to pump out to the body. When this happens, blood can pool in the chambers. When blood pools, blood clots can form. These blood clots can travel anywhere in the body, cause blockages, and create problems. When they travel to the brain, they can cause a stroke. In people who have strokes, 15–20% have AF (American Heart Association, 2014).

Sometimes cardiac disease is beyond the person's control or may be something the person is predisposed to. For example, some people are born with heart defects. If there is a history of cardiac disease in a family, the chances of having heart disease is increased. Age is another uncontrollable factor. As you get older, your risk increases; this is especially true for women whose risk increases after the age of 55 (National Heart, Lung, and Blood Institute, 2014).

Taking medications as directed by their doctor, eating a "heart healthy" diet, exercising regularly, and quitting smoking are some proven ways to help manage and/or prevent cardiac diseases. Having heart disease can be very frightening for a person who may feel that they could have a heart attack at any moment, so your caregivee/loved one will need supportive and gentle care.

The daily activities of a person with a cardiac illness may sometimes become limited. The severity of the heart disease may determine how much activity your caregivee/loved one can enjoy. Previously "routine" activities may be limited. Talk with the doctor, nurse, or health care team about daily activities, recreation, leisure activities, and sex. Some people may believe that exercise will "hurt" rather than help their condition, but some kinds of moderate exercise can help strengthen the heart, improve circulation, and lower blood pressure. In general, the exercises allowed may be limited to walking, cycling, and swimming. Your caregivee/loved one's doctor and health care team are the experts on your caregivee/loved one's unique heart and health problems. Ask them for any specific information and recommendations for care.

You may refer to other chapters in this book such as: "Bed-bound Care (Care of the Immobilized or Bedridden Patient)," "Stroke Care (Cerebrovascular Accident)," "Chronic Obstructive Pulmonary (COPD) Care," "Diabetes Care," "End-of-Life Care," and "Older Adult Care."

2. General Information: Symptoms of a heart attack may include pain in the arm and/or neck or chest area, nausea, dizziness and shortness of breath.

If your caregivee/loved one has had a heart attack, they may have had heart surgery or other procedures to make the blood flow better to the heart. After a heart attack, your caregivee/loved one will need ongoing special care because even though they have received treatment, the heart may have been damaged during the heart attack. And they will need to manage their "risk factors" more closely. After a heart attack, your caregivee/loved one may have spent time in the hospital. They may have had a procedure, such as an angioplasty (a procedure to increase circulation to the heart muscle) and/or they may have had a "stent" placed to keep blood vessels open to help blood flow to the heart. While in the hospital they may have learned how to take their pulse (heart rate), how to measure their blood pressure, and how to recognize angina (chest pain) and what to do if it occurs. Most commonly, the chest pain associated with heart attacks involves discomfort in the center or left side of the chest. The discomfort/pain may feel like nausea or indigestion. It may be mild or it may be severe. It generally lasts for more than a few minutes, and it can also go away and come back. It may be described as "tightness," "pressure," or "fullness." There may be pain in one or both arms, the shoulders, the neck, or the jaw. The person having a heart attack may complain of stomach pain just above their belly button. The doctor may have given your caregivee/loved one an exercise test and made recommendations about how much and what type of exercises to do at home. Medications are often prescribed after a heart attack as well. The doctor may prescribe anti-platelet drugs often known as "blood thinners," ACE-inhibitors (to reduce blood pressure), and/or "statin" drugs to help reduce cholesterol. You will find more information about medications commonly used to treat various heart conditions further on in this chapter.

Older people may sometimes have heart disease as a result of a general weakening of the heart muscle. This is known as heart failure, or CHF. CHF is compounded by other health issues, such as immobility, COPD (which is a serious respiratory condition), and/or kidney disease. CHF typically causes the symptoms of difficulty breathing, especially when lying flat and/or swelling of the legs, arms and abdomen, or "belly." CHF is sometimes treated with medications that may require frequent dosage changes ordered by the doctor. A sudden change is unusual in a person with CHF; if they experience chest pain, call the doctor or 911 right away. It is best to call your caregivee/loved one's doctor, nurse, or health care team at the first sign of a problem.

Managing CHF on a daily basis may help prevent an emergency department visit or hospitalization. For most people, CHF is a chronic or long-term condition and it cannot be cured. CHF can be managed and treated so that your caregivee/loved one can live an enjoyable life. As a caregiver, you will learn to recognize common early signs of a problem and work with your caregivee/loved one's doctor, nurse, or health care team to treat the symptoms, which may help prevent serious complications. Daily activities may be harder to perform because the heart is not pumping as well as it should.

People with an irregular heart rate and rhythm known as "A Fib" or AF, may or may not have symptoms such as chest pain, but even without symptoms, AF can lead to stroke. AF can happen every now and again or it may be a long-term condition. People with AF can live normal, healthy lives and for some people, medications can restore normal heart rhythms. People who have permanent AF may be able to control symptoms and prevent complications with treatments that include medications, medical procedures, medical devices, and lifestyle changes. Signs and symptoms of AF include "palpitations" or a sense that the heart is "fluttering." Chest pain, dizziness, shortness of breath, feeling fatigued, and feeling weak may all occur. Confusion and anxiety are also signs and symptoms of AF. The two most common complications that can result from AF are stroke and heart failure. In some individuals with AF, anticoagulants are also used to decrease the risk of embolic stroke.

Medications may be used to slow the heart rate down. These medications may be called beta-blockers and/or calcium channel blockers. A medication known as digitalis or digoxin may be prescribed and there are other medications that may be used as well. Work closely with your caregivee/loved one and establish a good "line of communication" with the doctor, nurse, or health care team.

Medications used to treat heart ailments often require close and frequent monitoring. Your caregivee/loved one may have a medication regimen that is tailored just for them. Always follow the doctor's instructions regarding medications and blood tests. Your caregivee/loved one may be on "blood thinning" medication to lessen the chance of a blood clot forming. If this is the case, and depending on the medications and doctors' instructions, they will usually need regular blood tests to make sure the blood is not too thin or too thick. It is important to keep all appointments for blood work. These test results should be given to the doctor so that they may make dosage changes as needed. Keeping a log and using a calendar is a good idea. Write down any blood test results and medication changes as well as any symptoms on this calendar. Have it handy if you call the doctor and bring it with you to doctor's appointments. You will want to watch for signs of bleeding since this may happen if the blood becomes too thin. Signs of bleeding may show up as bruises under the skin; bleeding gums; or black, sticky tar-like stools. If you see any of these signs of bleeding, call the doctor, nurse, or health care team right away. Be especially cautious if your caregivee/loved one experiences a fall and monitor them closely for signs and symptoms of bleeding. Always call the doctor if your caregivee/loved one falls.

Some cardiac caregivee/loved ones have a medical device implanted in their chest which makes the heart beat at a normal rate and rhythm. This device is called a pacemaker. Another device that some people receive is called an "implanted defibrillator." This device can detect an irregular heart beat and stimulate the heart back to a regular rate and rhythm. The doctor will have worked closely with your caregivee/loved one to decide on the best type of device to use. Pacemakers and/or implanted defibrillators are small, metal devices that contain a battery and a generator. They are placed just under the skin and are located on the chest wall. You will read more about pacemakers and implanted defibrillators later in this chapter.

3. General Goals for Care: Bottom line goals: Recognize common early symptoms of a heart attack (CAD), heart failure (CHF), or atrial fibrillation (AF) and help with the current management of your caregivee/loved one's condition.

If quick action is taken during a heart attack, further damage to the heart muscle might not occur. Once a person has had a heart attack, they are at higher risk to have a second heart attack. The symptoms of a second heart attack may or may not be the same symptoms that the person experienced with their first heart attack. It is important to make a plan to deal with a heart attack before it happens. Learn to recognize the warning signs of a heart attack, which may include chest pain or discomfort, upper body discomfort, and shortness of breath. A person having a heart attack may have crushing chest pain, but it is very important to note that someone having a heart attack does not always have chest pain. People who are older, female, and/or those with diabetes are known to sometimes have heart attacks without chest pain. Most commonly, the chest pain associated with heart attacks involves discomfort in the center or left side of the chest. The discomfort/pain may feel like nausea or indigestion. It may be mild or it may be severe. It generally lasts for more than a few minutes, and it can also go away and come back. It may be described as "tightness," "pressure," or "fullness." There may be pain in one or both arms, the shoulders, the neck, or the jaw. The person having a heart attack may complain of stomach pain just above their belly button. Shortness of breath may be an early warning sign and it may occur when the person is at rest or with a small amount of activity. Chest pain that doesn't go away and/or that happens with increasing frequency or, for example, while a person is resting, may be a sign of a heart attack. Sometimes, people who have had a heart attack have the same symptoms again. All chest pain should be checked by the doctor.

Your caregivee/loved one may have been told that they have "angina." Angina is chest pain, pressure, or a squeezing feeling in the chest. It is a symptom of an underlying heart problem. It is not a heart attack, but it does mean that a heart attack is more likely to happen in the future. Your caregivee/ loved one may have had a medication such as Nitroglycerin prescribed to take when they are experiencing an episode of angina. There are two types of angina: stable and unstable. Stable angina tends to occur in a pattern and it happens when the heart is working harder than usual. Stable angina can sometimes be anticipated and avoided. The caregivee/ loved one may have been directed by their doctor to take medication before engaging in an activity such as bathing or walking. With stable angina, the pain usually goes away after the caregivee/loved one has rested and/or taken their angina medication. Unstable angina does not follow a pattern and the pain can be more severe than with stable angina. It may not be brought on by exertion and the pain may not be relieved with rest or after taking medication. Unstable angina is serious and may be an indicator that a heart attack is going to happen. People who are experiencing chest pain should immediately rest and take their prescribed chest pain medication if one has been ordered by the doctor. Chest pain should always be evaluated—when in doubt call 911!

After a heart attack, your caregivee/loved one may have been advised to make changes to their lifestyles that may prevent another heart attack in the future. A "heart healthy" diet, maintaining a healthy weight, regular exercise, and quitting smoking may have been recommended. Your caregivee/loved one may have been prescribed medication to help chest pain, lower cholesterol, and/or to treat high blood pressure. The doctor may have recommended a cardiac rehabilitation program, often called "cardiac rehab." Cardiac rehab is a medically supervised program that helps with the health and well being of a person after they have had a heart attack. Cardiac rehab also helps a person learn to deal with stress and depression. Cardiac rehab units are often staffed by a team of health care professionals and may include your caregivee/loved one's family doctor as well as cardiac doctors, surgeons, nurses, dietitians, physical therapists, and counselors. Cardiac rehab usually requires a long-term commitment from your caregivee/loved one and may be very beneficial.

Not all people who have had a heart attack are able to exercise. If your caregivee/loved one has very high blood pressure or has suffered severe heart damage, they might not be able to participate in the exercise portion of a cardiac rehabilitation program.

For a person with CHF, the goal is to know what can be done to improve and maintain the heart's "pumping power." Your caregivee/loved one may experience some of the following symptoms if they are struggling with CHF: difficulty breathing (especially when lying down flat); difficulty with daily activities; swollen ankles, feet, legs or belly/abdomen; weight gain; a frequent dry and hacking cough; and waking up feeling breathless and/or waking up feeling tired and/or anxious, confused, or disoriented.

The condition of a person with CHF can worsen if prescribed medications are skipped. Always refill the medications so that your caregivee/loved one does not run out, and follow the doctor's directions. The medications that your caregivee/ loved one may be prescribed are the following: ACE Inhibitors are medications that make it easier for the heart to pump, Vasodilators help open up the blood vessels (dilation) to lower blood pressure, Diuretics (or "water pills") help remove salt and excess water or fluid from the body, Digitalis medications strengthen each heartbeat and help the heart beat more effectively, Beta Blockers generally decrease the heart's beating rate if it is going too fast, and/or Calcium Channel Blockers can be used to improve circulation and lower blood pressure. As noted on a prior page, the caregivee/loved one might be on blood thinners and they may also be on statin drugs, which are used to decrease cholesterol.

A heart healthy diet is important for everyone to help decrease the risk of heart disease, and is an especially important approach for people who have heart disease. A heart healthy diet has decreased salt and decreased saturated fat and cholesterol. Salt, or sodium, causes fluid to build up in the body, and this fluid buildup causes the heart to work harder. Too much salt also causes arteries to thicken which can lead to decreased blood flow to the heart. Examples of high salt or high sodium foods are: canned soups, dry soup mixes, canned meats and fish, bacon, ham, sausage, butter, margarine, and packaged frozen dinners. Saturated fats are fats that cause cholesterol levels to rise. Cholesterol is the waxy/fatty deposits, sometimes called "plaque," that can line the blood vessels, causing atherosclerosis. Limiting foods such as red meats, butter, dairy products, eggs, shortening, lard, and palm and coconut oils will decrease the saturated fats in your diet. Any fat that is not liquid at room temperature should be avoided. Fast foods are often high in sodium and saturated fats and should be limited or avoided. Drinks containing alcohol decrease the heart's ability to contract and should be eliminated or limited to one drink two to three times a week. "One drink" means one small glass of wine, one beer, or 1 ounce of alcohol in a mixed drink. Caffeine can act as a heart stimulant, causing stress on the heart. Try to limit or eliminate caffeine in the diet. Juice and water are always better choices. Only use salt substitutes if recommended by the doctor. Use low salt seasonings such as lemon juice and herbs. Fresh vegetables are always best, but frozen vegetables are available year round and low-sodium canned fruits and vegetables are available.

4. Personal Care Considerations: People with cardiac disease may be less active, especially in the time period just after or following a heart attack. Following a heart attack, the heart needs to rest and heal. Ask the doctor, nurse, or health care team what activities the person is allowed to engage in, and what activities to avoid. The doctor may limit exercise at first and then gradually increase the amount of exercise over time. Any increase in activity, different than what the doctor, nurse, or health care team has recommended, should be approved by them first.

Your caregivee/loved one may be advised to limit household tasks that used to be "routine." Some people with heart disease will be tired and need frequent rest periods between tasks. As caregiver, you may notice shortness of breath, which may mean your caregivee/loved one needs a rest period. They may have been prescribed medication to address angina, such as Nitroglycerin. If your caregivee/loved one becomes short of breath, complains of being tired, and/or has angina, have them sit down and give them their medication as directed. Keep this medication handy at all times. Nitroglycerin may have a short "shelf life," so check the date on the medicine bottle to make sure that the medication will be ready when you need it. Continue with the care you are providing only after your caregivee/loved one has told you he/she is ready to do so. As always, explain what you are going to do and what you are doing, as you do it.

If your caregivee/loved one has CHF, they may have swelling in their legs. They may wear special hose or stockings. Many people with CHF need to keep their legs up as much as possible in order to reduce stress on the heart. Sudden changes in symptoms of persons with CHF are not expected. If your caregivee/loved one has been prescribed nitroglycerin for angina, they may have been instructed to take it before they start a strenuous activity. If your caregivee/loved one complains of angina, it is best to have them stop the activity, sit down, and take their nitroglycerin as prescribed. Call the doctor or 911 if the chest pain continues after the medication has been given. Also call 911 if there is an increase in the frequency or severity of the pain.

Persons with CHF need to monitor their diet closely. Too much sodium in the diet can cause fluid buildup and the person's feet, ankles, and abdomen may swell. This swelling can cause difficulty breathing. If swelling and/or difficulty breathing becomes severe, the doctor, nurse, or health care team should be contacted. The doctor might make changes to the medication routine. To help your caregivee/loved one reduce their salt intake you might remove the salt shaker from the eating table and from the stove area.

Periods of rest are very important for the person with CHF.

It is important for them to sit down often and elevate their feet and legs, perhaps on a foot stool or in a recliner chair. This action relieves stress on the heart. It is important to do this after meals.

If your caregivee/loved one has CHF they may be on a "fluid restricted" diet. If this is the case, they will need to monitor how much fluid they drink in a day. Record the amount of fluid that your caregivee/loved one drinks in each 24 hour period. It is good to remember that 1 cup equals 8 ounces. Starting a log, perhaps using a calendar page, will be very helpful. This information will help the doctor, nurse, or health care team member to make any necessary adjustments in their treatment plan. Your caregivee/loved one may be taking a diuretic medication or "water pill." This will help to remove excess fluid from the body and reduce stress on the heart. This medication may cause a person to urinate more frequently. Usually, diuretics are taken in the morning so that your caregivee/loved one can experience a good night's sleep. The fluid that the caregivee/loved one is eliminating does not need to be replaced. This medication may make them experience a dry mouth. If this is the case, sucking on hard candy or ice chips may alleviate dry mouth without adding unwanted fluid back into the body.

A caregivee/loved one with CHF will need to watch their weight closely. Any fluid buildup in the body will show in their weight. Have an accurate bathroom scale that your caregivee/loved one can access safely. Weigh them every morning, after urinating but before eating. Always use the same scale on the same floor. Record the weight every morning in your caregivee/loved one's log or notebook. In general, if they gain two pounds or more overnight or five pounds or more in a week, you should call their doctor, nurse, or health care team right away. The doctor may have given you other guidelines and, if so, follow them. If the doctor, nurse, or health care team has not given you guidelines, we strongly urge you to ask them!

Keep track of other symptoms in your caregivee/loved one's log or notebook as well, such as episodes of chest pain and/or shortness of breath. It is a good idea to monitor swelling in the feet and ankles. If your caregivee/loved one's ankles are swollen, gently push against the skin with a finger. If it remains indented, this is a sign of edema, or fluid buildup, and should be recorded on your caregivee/loved one's log and reported to the doctor, nurse, or health care team. Always report changes in your caregivee/loved one's condition. Gradually, over time, you will learn what is "normal" and what is a change. When you call the doctor, nurse, or health care team, have your caregivee/loved one's log or notebook handy to refer to and be sure to state that you are calling about a person who is being treated for heart failure. Be sure to keep all doctor appointments.

People with heart disease may tire easily or experience shortness of breath. It will be important for them to conserve energy as much as possible. As caregiver, you can help by making rest periods an everyday "activity." Eating small, frequent meals; avoiding stressful people and situations; and avoiding people who have a cold or influenza (flu) are all ways that you and your caregivee/loved one may conserve energy. Place chairs throughout the house for your caregivee/loved one to sit on and rest. Have them move slowly and sit when performing routine tasks. It is important not to slow the blood flow to the legs. Tight stockings and shoes should be avoided. Wearing loose clothing can also help with comfort and conserving energy.

If your caregivee/loved one has a pacemaker, they should avoid prolonged exposure to electrical devices or devices with a strong magnetic field such as: electrical generators, microwave ovens, metal detectors, or high tension wires. Prolonged exposure can disrupt the effectiveness of the pacemaker. The caregivee/loved one may not know if the pacemaker has been effected. The risk of the pacemaker being effected depends upon how long the pacemaker is exposed to the device that has the magnetic field, and how strong the magnetic field is. Pacemakers have features built in to protect them against these strong magnetic fields, but awareness and caution should guide you. It is safe to use a microwave oven and other household appliances, but prolonged exposure should be minimized. Always check with your caregivee/loved one's doctor about their specific device and any safety recommendations. When in doubt, ask! Some medical tests and procedures such as an MRI machine can disrupt a pacemaker. Be sure to let all doctors and dentists know that your caregivee has a pacemaker or other implanted device. Have your caregivee/loved one carry their pacemaker/defibrillator identification (ID) card with them at all times.

Having regular bowel movements may seem like a small thing, but it is actually a very large part of a person's comfort. This is especially relevant for a person with cardiac disease. Straining to pass a bowel movement can be very taxing on the heart. If your caregivee/loved one is on any pain medication, it is very likely it can and will cause constipation. Sometimes stool softener or laxatives are prescribed to prevent straining during bowel movements.

5. Safety Considerations: When scheduling a dentist appointment, always let the dentist know that your caregivee/loved one has had cardiac issues. If your caregivee/loved one has an implanted device such as a pacemaker or defibrillator, they will have been given an ID card that identifies the specific type of device that they have. They should carry this ID card with them at all times. The dentist should also be told if your caregivee/loved one is on blood thinning medications. Ask the dentist if there is oxygen available in case of an emergency. If your caregivee/loved one takes Nitroglycerin or another rescue medication for angina, be sure that they have it with them and can access it.

Know how to react to chest pain when it happens. Have your caregivee/loved one sit, stay calm, and rest. As caregiver, it is very important that you remain calm as well and provide a calm environment. Suggest that your caregivee/loved one breathe deeply and slowly. If they take Nitroglycerin, administer it exactly as directed. Allow Nitroglycerin to dissolve under the tongue—do not swallow it. Have your caregivee/loved one sit down when they take their Nitroglycerin. Keep a record of when chest pain or other cardiac episode, such as lightheadedness or dizziness, occurred. Write down the time of day and what your caregivee/loved one was doing when the event occurred. Write down what helped or did not help the situation. Write down what the pain felt like and how long it lasted. Was your caregivee/loved one more active than normal? Had they taken their medications as prescribed? Write this information on their log and bring it with you to doctor's appointments and/or to the emergency department. Bring the caregivee/loved one's medication bottles to all doctor's appointments, including over-the-counter medications and any medications prescribed by other doctors. Bring them to the emergency department as well. When you call the doctor, nurse, or health care team, have the log/notebook handy to refer to and be sure to state that you are calling about a person who is being treated for a heart condition.

Your caregivee/loved one may need to avoid specific activities that strain the heart, such as walking uphill, walking up stairs, or shoveling. Avoid temperature extremes. Angina often occurs in cold weather. The doctor may have prescribed medication to be taken before any strenuous activity. Follow these instructions.

6. When to Call the Doctor, Nurse, or Care Team:

- Caregivee/loved one feels nauseated, dizzy, is short of breath, breaks out in cold sweat, or is experiencing chest pain five minutes after taking rescue medicine such as Nitroglycerin.
- Caregivee/loved one is feeling unusually tired for no reason, or having anxiety or other symptoms (especially if caregivee/loved one is a woman).
- Caregivee/loved one experiences lightheadedness or sudden dizziness that is unrelieved by sitting down.
- Caregivee/loved one experiences sudden weight gain of two pounds overnight or five pounds in one week's time.
- Caregivee/loved one experiences any sudden, new symptoms or a change in the pattern of symptoms they already have. Symptoms become stronger or last longer than usual.
- Caregivee/loved one has distressful nausea or nausea that won't go away, with or without vomiting.

- Caregivee/loved one has stopped eating or drinking or has difficulty swallowing.
- Caregivee/loved one has a change in how they urinate. Perhaps they cannot urinate or they are urinating much more frequently than usual, but only producing small amounts of urine. Perhaps their urine has changed color, is very dark, and/or has a strong odor.
- Caregivee/loved one has had a change in their bowel movements or has stopped having bowel movements for more than three days, even if they are not eating very much.
- Caregivee/loved one is very emotional, perhaps they cannot stop crying or they are showing other obvious signs of distress. Perhaps they are questioning their spiritual beliefs, or doubting what they once believed.
- Caregivee/loved one has fallen.
- Caregivee/loved one has shortness of breath that does not go away after the usual measures are taken to alleviate it.
- Caregivee/loved one has a cough that produces white or blood tinged sputum.
- Caregivee/loved one is wheezing.
- Caregivee/loved one has a higher or faster heart rate than usual that is unrelieved after resting for five minutes.
- Caregivee/loved one has unexplained bruising or larger bruises than you would normally expect.
- Caregivee/loved one has a sudden or high fever.
- Caregivee/loved one cannot get comfortable/find relief from pain. For example, pain wakes caregivee/loved one up at night or pain comes on suddenly. Always believe whatever your caregivee/loved one tells you about their pain. Caregivee/loved ones are the expert on their pain.

- Caregivee/loved one has white spots or a white coating on their tongue, or any other kind of mouth sore.
- Any other change, complication or concern that you or the caregivee/loved one may have. When in doubt, call!

These are examples only. Your caregivee/loved one might relay to you changes or concerns that vary from those listed here and those concerns should be addressed with your care team.

7. Comfort Considerations: Comfort for your caregivee/loved one can mean physical, mental, spiritual, or any combination of those kinds of comfort. As a caregiver, providing comfort sometimes means "the small things." Small things are sometimes easily overlooked.

Straining during a bowel movement is very taxing on the heart. Sometimes the person may need to take a stool softener or laxative daily. Please ask the doctor, nurse, or health care team about this. If your caregivee/loved one is on any pain medication, they can and, in many cases, do cause constipation. Unfortunately, sometimes your health care team may forget to tell you this! It is always better to prevent a problem than to correct a problem, and this is never more true than when it comes to pain medicines and constipation. We encourage you not to be shy about asking your caregivee/loved one about their bowel habits and call the doctor or clinic if their bowels have not moved for three days. This is true even if they are not eating very much and is important to remember for caregivee/loved ones with cardiac disease.

Sometimes distraction, such as watching TV or a movie,

reading, or playing cards is enough to ease a person's anxiety. Spending time with a beloved pet is often a wonderful therapy, particularly for those who are feeling emotionally "down" or depressed. A visit to their place of worship, from a member of their church, or to a place that is spiritually meaningful to your caregivee/loved one, such as a drive to the ocean, may comfort them spiritually. As always, your caregivee/loved one will often be the best person to guide you in what they need.

Some persons with cardiac disease may be using oxygen therapy. Supplemental oxygen might help prevent weakness, dizziness, and shortness of breath as well as the anxiety that people experience when they feel they are not getting enough air. Oxygen should be considered a very important comfort measure. Oxygen is a drug and the amount to be received is prescribed by the doctor. Use it only as prescribed. All combustible materials should be removed from the area and no open flames or candles can be used in the room! NEVER smoke while on oxygen because serious facial and internal burns to the mouth and throat can occur. Smoking is prohibited in areas where oxygen is used for good reason.

Your caregivee/loved one may experience difficulty sleeping at night. They may experience shortness of breath and/ or coughing when they lie flat. Naps during the daytime may help if your caregivee/loved one is feeling tired from a lack of sleep. Using more than one pillow to prop the head up may help them sleep better. Keeping the head and chest elevated by raising the mattress from underneath may also be helpful. The doctor, nurse, or health care team may suggest a foam "wedge" to lay on or to position under their mattress to help them to breathe better when lying down.

Sometimes your caregivee/loved one may ask to be left alone for a while. Please don't take this personally! Living with cardiac disease disrupts a person's whole life, and it affects those around them, including and, perhaps especially, the caregiver. Give your caregivee/loved one time to "regroup" if they ask for it, and use this time to do something nice for yourself. If your caregivee/loved one doesn't recover from their need to be alone after a day or two, it's time to talk to them about it, and very possibly time to call the doctor or clinic.

A clean fresh mouth helps a person feel comfortable and may head off problems of the mouth at an early stage. Sometimes, illness and their treatments can put a person at risk for mouth sores or a fungal infection in the mouth called "thrush." Notify the doctor, nurse, or health care team if your caregivee/loved one develops any mouth problems or changes. People with cardiac disease may have difficulty raising their arms up to brush their teeth. It may be helpful to have the person sit to perform personal care to reduce stress on the heart. A chair in the bathroom or near the kitchen sink may be very helpful.

People with heart disease can feel anxious and depressed. They may feel fearful performing daily tasks that were once routine and they may be grieving for how they lived before their illness. These feelings may subside over time as the person experiences an adjustment period. Allow them to go at their own pace as much as possible. Try to be an active listener. An active listener quietly listens to the person's fears and experiences without interrupting. Allow your caregivee/loved one to draw their own conclusions, even if they sound sad or you do not agree. Your caregivee/loved one may express a range of emotions as they adjust to their new lifestyle. With time, your caregivee/loved one can find the pace and lifestyle that accommodates them comfortably.

8. Special Considerations: If your caregivee/loved one's heart or breathing stops and you call 911, medical care and treatment will be provided. Sometimes this treatment is quite aggressive. If your caregivee/loved one is an older person, they may want to speak with their doctor, if they have not done so already, about *advanced directives*. Advanced directives let caregivers, doctors, and emergency personnel know what the person's wishes are if they can no longer speak for themselves. Specific instructions, such as do not resuscitate, regarding their wishes may be needed in the event of a medical emergency. For more information and resources related to this topic please refer to the chapters entitled "End-of-Life Care" and "Older Adult Care."

9. Special Instructions Given to You by the Doctor, Nurse, or Care Team:

_____

_____

_____

_____

_____

_____

_____

_____

_____

10. Resources:

- The National Institute on Aging offers a "Heart Health" resource on their AgePage: http://www.nia.nih.gov/health/publication/heart-health?utm_source=20150209_hearthealth&utm_medium=email&utm_campaign=ealert
- The American Heart Association offers information on their website about heart attacks and stroke, including "Heart and Stroke Statistics": http://www.heart.org/HEARTORG/General/Heart-and-Stroke-Association-Statistics_UCM_319064_SubHomePage.jsp?utm_campaign=statistics&utm_source=cvdstroke&utm_medium=newsletter
- The American Heart Association also offers information about "Caregiver Responsibility": http://www.heart.org/HEARTORG/Caregiver/Responsibilities/ResponsibilityIntroduction/Caregiver-Responsibility-Introduction_UCM_301828_Article.jsp
- The Centers for Disease Control and Prevention (CDC) offers information about heart disease on their Heart Disease Facts page: http://www.cdc.gov/heartdisease/facts.htm
- The Health Resources and Services Administration offers information about amputation through their Lower Extremity Amputation Prevention (LEAP) program's site: http://www.hrsa.gov/hansensdisease/leap/

References

American Heart Association. (2014). What is Atrial Fibrillation (AFib or AF)? Retrieved from http://www.heart.org/HEARTORG/Conditions/Arrhythmia/AboutArrhythmia/What-is-Atrial-Fibrillation-AFib-or-AF_UCM_423748_Article.jsp

Centers for Disease Control and Prevention (CDC). (2015). "Heart Disease Facts." Retrieved from http://www.cdc.gov/heartdisease/facts.htm

Centers for Disease Control and Prevention (CDC). (2012). "NCHS Data Brief: Hospitalization for Congestive Heart Failure: United States, 2000–2010." Retrieved from http://www.cdc.gov/nchs/data/databriefs/db108.htm

National Heart, Lung, and Blood Institute. (2013). "Who Is at Risk for Heart Disease?" Retrieved from http://www.nhlbi.nih.gov/health/health-topics/topics/hdw/atrisk

National Heart, Lung, and Blood Institute. (2013). "What Causes a Heart Attack?" Retrieved from http://www.nhlbi.nih.gov/health/health-topics/topics/heartattack/causes

CHRONIC OBSTRUCTIVE PULMONARY DISEASE (COPD) CARE

1. Introduction: Chronic Obstructive Pulmonary Disease (COPD) is a long-term lung disease in which the lung's airways become obstructed and this condition causes difficulty breathing. COPD is also sometimes called Chronic Obstructive Airway Disease and/or Chronic Obstructive Lung Disease. You may also hear the term "pulmonary" to describe the lungs, and sometimes these words are used interchangeably. COPD is a progressive disease, which means it gets worse over time. COPD can cause a productive cough, which is a cough that produces mucus. COPD can cause wheezing, shortness of breath, and a tight feeling in the chest. COPD usually refers to the diseases emphysema and/or chronic bronchitis. Often, a person with COPD will have both of these diseases, but COPD is not limited to just emphysema and chronic bronchitis. Smoking is the primary cause of COPD and people who have been exposed long-term to other air pollutants, chemical fumes, or dusts can develop COPD. According to a study performed by the National Institute of Health between 1999 and 2011, 13.7 million adults over the age of 25 were diagnosed with COPD (Ford et al., 2013). In 2010, COPD resulted in 10.3 million doctor's office visits, 1.5 million emergency room visits, and 133,575 deaths (Ford et al., 2013). You will find more COPD-specific resources listed at the end of this chapter.

COPD is not a curable disease, but it is a disease that can

be managed. If you learn as much as possible about this disease and work closely with your caregivee/loved one's doctor, nurse, or health care team, it is possible to maintain an enjoyable life and help receive timely treatment to prevent complications that could lead to visits to the emergency department and/or hospitalizations.

You may also refer to other chapters in this book such as: "Cardiac Care," "End-of-Life Care," and "Older Adult Care."

2. General Information: The lungs are part of the body's respiratory system, the system in the body that provides oxygen to the blood. Understanding how the respiratory system works will help you and your caregivee/loved one to better manage this illness. For information on the anatomy and physiology of the respiratory system, visit "The Respiratory System" page from the National Heart, Lung, and Blood Institute: http://www.nhlbi.nih.gov/health/health-topics/topics/hlw/system. You may also find the video animation entitled "What is COPD?" from the National Heart, Lung, and Blood Institute helpful: https://www.youtube.com/watch?v=BIdHQQEXPDk.

The lung tissue contains tiny elasticized sacks that take oxygen in and exchange it for carbon dioxide. We breathe oxygen in and carbon dioxide out. This is referred to as "air exchange." In a person living with COPD, the lung tissue has lost its elasticity and is unable to effectively make that exchange. Mucus, a slippery substance that the body naturally produces, is often present in the lungs of caregivee/loved ones who have COPD. When the lungs have lost their elasticity and/or become filled with mucus, the person who has COPD may have difficulty breathing. Mucus can be a breeding ground for infections and, because of this, persons with COPD may be at increased risk to lung infections.

COPD occurs gradually, over time, and it is not contagious. You cannot catch it from another person. Usually, COPD is diagnosed in middle to older age adults and the symptoms of COPD do not typically show up until approximately age 40 or later. With careful management and attention to medications, treatment regimens, and lifestyle changes person may be able to control symptoms and have a satisfying and enjoyable quality of life.

Asthma can sometimes contribute to COPD. Acute asthma is not a cause of COPD, but uncontrolled chronic asthma may be. There is also a rare genetic form of emphysema, known as alpha-1 antitrypsin deficiency, that can cause COPD at an early age. Smoking or a history of smoking is the number one cause of COPD.

When a person first develops COPD, there are usually no symptoms. When symptoms do develop they may include a cough with or without mucus, a tight feeling in the chest, and/or shortness of breath noticed with exertion such as walking up stairs. Not everyone with these symptoms has COPD. A person with COPD notices that the symptoms increase over time and they start to make adjustments to accommodate the disease, such as taking the elevator instead of the stairs. Over time, the symptoms may become severe enough that the person needs to see a doctor, and this may be when COPD is diagnosed. Unfortunately, the more severe the symptoms are, the more lung damage is indicated. Advanced, or severe, COPD can cause symptoms such as swelling of the feet and ankles, weight loss, and muscle wasting, a condition in which the muscles become thin and weak. The doctor diagnoses COPD based on signs and symptoms; the person's medical, family, and work history; and through lung function tests. To learn more about specific lung function tests visit: http://www.nhlbi.nih.gov/health/health-topics/topics/lft/. Lung function tests usually do not cause pain and are not invasive. The doctor may be checking the person's cardiac (heart) status when they check the lung function. This is because the heart and lungs are closely related and what affects one, affects the other. For more information on the anatomy and physiology of the heart, visit "How the Heart Works" from the National Heart, Lung, and Blood Institute: http://www.nhlbi.nih.gov/health/health-topics/topics/hhw.

The symptoms of a person with COPD due to chronic bronchitis may include: a long-term or perhaps persistent cough, increased mucus production, shortness of breath, and frequent clearing of the throat. If your caregivee/loved one has emphysema, their symptoms may include: cough or shortness of breath. Both illnesses can lead to a limited ability to engage in physical exercise.

Because persons who have COPD are at increased risk for getting colds, flu (influenza), and respiratory infections, your caregivee/loved one may have recurrent episodes of bronchitis or pneumonia. Persons with COPD may be on a care regimen that includes oxygen therapy, medications, inhalers, and exercise programs. It is likely that they will have been advised to stop smoking. If they have not already, they should stop smoking! It is important that persons with COPD adhere to their care program and avoid infections, which can lead to hospitalizations.

3. General Goals for Care: Bottom line goals: prevent disease progression, support optimal air exchange, and prevent infections. These goals may be achieved by following recommendations about diet, medications, and other habits.

To prevent disease progression, the underlying cause of the illness needs to be addressed. If your caregivee/loved one smokes, it's time to quit. If someone in their environment smokes, it is time for them to quit or to "take it outside." It has been said that second hand smoke is like smoking without a filter for everyone else in the room. In addition, second hand smoke has been linked to childhood asthma, ear infections in children, and upper respiratory illnesses in children. COPD cannot be cured, but it's progression can be slowed. Reduce exposure to both indoor and outdoor air pollution by avoiding dust; household chemicals; personal care aerosols; and outdoor smoke, fumes, and vapors.

Your caregivee/loved one's doctor may have prescribed medication, oxygen, and breathing exercises to help maximize their breathing efforts. It is important to remember that finding the correct medication, dosage, and schedule may take time. We encourage you to maintain open, healthy communication with your caregivee/loved one's health care team. Medications can cause side effects and these should be reported right away. The caregivee/loved one should always take the correct dose of their medication at the right time as prescribed by the doctor. No medication should be stopped and no medication doses should be changed without speaking with the doctor first. Tell the doctor about all medications your caregivee/loved one is taking, including over-the-counter medications and vitamins and supplements. Some cough medications suppress a cough, but it is likely that the doctor will want the caregivee/loved one to expel mucus rather than quell a cough, so please check before taking any over-the-counter cough medications. And always bring all medications with you to your caregivee/loved one's doctor's appointments, including medications prescribed by other physicians.

Some medications that may be prescribed for persons with COPD are: antibiotics if the caregivee/loved one has an infection or bronchodilators to open airways and allow air to move in and out of the respiratory system more easily. Bronchodilators may cause a person to feel nervous or "jittery" and they may interfere with sleep. Let the doctor, nurse, or health care team know if this is happening. Diuretics, sometimes called "water pills," may be given to remove excess fluid from the body. Excess fluid can make it hard to breathe. Diuretics can make people urinate more frequently, and are often taken in the morning to ensure an uninterrupted night's sleep. The fluid that is removed by a diuretic does not need to be replaced. Sometimes, when a person is on diuretics, they may need to take a potassium supplement. Ask the doctor, nurse, or health care team about this. They may recommend food that is potassium rich or the doctor may prescribe a potassium supplement. Some inhaled medications include directions to rinse the mouth after using; be sure to follow the directions. Your caregivee/loved one may be taking steroids to ease breathing and to help decrease swelling in the airways. The doctor may prescribe inhaled or oral steroids. No one should ever suddenly stop taking steroids! Steroids, if taken over a long period of time, can have serious side effects. One possible side effect is a weakened immune system. Be sure to monitor your caregivee/loved one for any type of infection. Prevent infection if at all possible.

Oxygen is another treatment that the doctor might prescribe for a person with COPD. Oxygen should be treated as a medication. It may be prescribed for use at night while sleeping, for use during periods of exercise, or continuously or intermittently as needed throughout the day. Oxygen is a vital comfort measure, but it is not curative. You will read more about the use of oxygen under safety considerations. There are several types of breathing devices that are used to deliver medication directly to the airways and lungs. These are often referred to as "breathing treatments" and will be shown to you and your caregivee/loved one by the doctor, nurse, or health care team. A respiratory therapist may be part of your health care team and they may show you how to perform breathing exercises prescribed by the doctor. Common devices may include multi-dose inhalers and/or nebulizer treatments. Multi-dose inhalers (MDIs) are sometimes called "puffers." You and your caregivee/loved one will have been shown how to use an MDI by the doctor, nurse, or health care team. It is good to remember to have the caregivee/loved one hold the medication in the lungs for 10 seconds if possible so that the medication can settle in and not be breathed out. Some inhalers have a short-term effect and others are used for long-term symptom management. Short-term inhalers may be prescribed to address a sudden onset of symptoms and/or they may be used as pre-medication prior to caregivee/loved one activities. Follow all instructions provided. Another type of device frequently prescribed to a person with COPD is a nebulizer. A nebulizer is a machine that turns liquid medication into a fine mist that is then inhaled into the lungs. The person may wear a mask over their nose and mouth or they may inhale it, as if from a "pipe." With both MDIs or nebulizers, the person should take their treatment while sitting upright. Some of these medications are used to clear mucus out of the lungs and airways.

Your doctor, nurse, or health care team member may have demonstrated coughing methods to help effectively clear mucus out of their respiratory system. It is important to clear out mucus not only to enhance breathing but also as a means of preventing infection. Mucus in the lungs can be a breeding ground for germs that can lead to infections such as a cold, acute bronchitis, or pneumonia. If mucus is produced, it is a good idea to note the color and thickness and report changes to the doctor, nurse, or health care team. If your caregivee/ loved one thinks that they would benefit by taking their nebulizer treatment more often than they have been advised to, discuss this with the prescriber or other health care team member. The nebulizer machine should be kept on a flat surface and the parts should be cleaned after every use. Follow the cleaning instructions that were shown to you and replace parts as instructed. Report any problems with the machine, such as leaking, to the company that provided it. Always stay "ahead of the game" and be proactive. If you see that the supply of equipment or medication needed to keep your caregivee/loved one comfortable is running low, call to order more before it runs out. Unfortunately, automated systems, such as voicemail, do not always run smoothly, so try to talk with a person directly to be sure your needs are addressed. It is better to avoid a problem than to address a problem, especially for a person who has breathing issues.

To prevent infection, it is important to keep breathing

devices clean. If your caregivee/loved one has COPD, it is best that they avoid inhaling strong household cleaners. Ask the doctor, nurse, or health care team members to recommend appropriate cleaning solutions for nebulizers and oxygen equipment. If oxygen is delivered by nasal prongs, called a nasal cannula, the nasal cannula should be changed at least every two weeks. The oxygen tubing itself and the humidifier bottle, if one is being used, should be changed at least every month, or as needed, or as directed by your health care team.

4. Personal Care Considerations: Preventing infection is very important for persons living with COPD, so hand washing before and after all personal care and food preparation is a must. Always let your caregivee/loved one know what you are going to do before you do it and what you are doing as you do it. A person with COPD may need to conserve energy throughout the day. They may feel most energized after a breathing treatment and that may be a good time to schedule care. It may be a good idea to ask the doctor if premedicating for shortness of breath prior to activities is a good idea. Plan ahead so that you can provide frequent rest periods during activities. Having chairs placed throughout the house for them to rest on may be helpful, as well as having chairs located in the kitchen and bathroom so they can sit to perform daily tasks. A shower chair in the bathroom may help conserve energy during bathing, or the caregivee/loved one may do better sitting for a sponge bath.

Your caregivee/loved one may become short of breath and frightened. If this happens, it is best that both you and your caregivee/loved one remain calm. Your caregivee/loved one may have become lightheaded from trying too hard to breathe. Have them sit down and, if the doctor has prescribed a "rescue dose" of any medication or has recommended using oxygen on an "as needed" basis, administer it. Never increase the oxygen flow amount without talking with the doctor; this could be very detrimental to the caregivee/loved one.

"Pursed lip breathing" is a breathing technique that may have been taught to your caregivee/loved one for when they feel they are not getting enough oxygen. They should relax, breath in slowly, and breathe out slowly, expelling the air through lips that are held in a whistling position. They should take twice the amount of time exhaling as they did to inhale. It is a good idea to practice pursed lip breathing several times a day so that it becomes a habit.

Your caregivee/loved one can conserve energy by scheduling rest periods every day. They may like to wait an hour after eating before engaging in activities because digesting food takes energy. Small, frequent meals are easier to digest than large meals. Using a small utility cart in the house to carry items from room to room is another way of conserving energy. Using a tray on a walker (sometimes called a walker tray) may also be helpful. Wearing less restrictive clothing, such as suspenders rather than belts and undershirts or camisoles instead of a bra, can allow for a feeling of easier air exchange. Using tongs or a "reacher" to pick up or retrieve items rather than bending may be helpful and a long-handled shoe horn is another energy conserving device.

Avoid individuals with colds or infections; all of these factors can cause tremendous stress on the body. Try to avoid crowds, especially during cold and influenza (flu) season. Persons living with COPD should use unscented deodorants and other grooming aids. Non-aerosol products are best because any inhaled substances can irritate the lungs. These can include powders and perfumes. Cold air can cause discomfort for a person with COPD and may make them feel short of breath. If you accompany your caregivee/loved one outdoors in a cold climate, have them breathe through their nose and consider using a cold weather mask, a scarf, or even their hand to cover their nose and mouth to avoid discomfort.

To help the person with COPD avoid infection, it is important that they keep their lungs as free of mucus as possible. Drinking plenty of fluids and eating a healthy diet can help with this. Drinking plenty of fluids helps to loosen the mucus in the lungs, making it thinner and easier to expel. A member of your caregivee/loved one's health care team may have shown you how to perform chest physiotherapy, or "chest PT." Chest PT can help clear mucus from the lungs. Chest PT uses positioning of the person and gravity to help drain mucus out of the lungs. If mucus cannot be expelled when the person coughs in their usual position, repositioning the person and using gravity to pull the mucus away from where it is resting may help. Having the person lie on one side rather than another or helping them move from a sitting position to a lying position may get the mucus moving. In addition to increased fluid intake and repositioning, you may have been shown how to cup your hand and pat the chest or vibrate the chest to loosen mucus from the chest walls. Once the mucus is loosened, it may be easier for the person to clear it from their lungs by coughing. If the doctor, nurse, or health care team has not shown you these techniques, ask them! If the doctor agrees that chest PT should be part of the treatment plan, you may find that early morning and before bedtime are good times to do it.

Coughing spells may make your caregivee/loved one feel tired and frightened, but coughing can be controlled. Coughing to clear mucus is beneficial. It is best to sit upright to cough, and have the person lean slightly forward. Have them breathe in deeply, if possible, when they feel a cough coming on. They should hold their breath for a few seconds and then cough out twice. The first cough will loosen the mucus and, with the second cough, they may be able to expel it. Use a tissue or paper towel to spit the mucus into and dispose of it immediately. Both you and your caregivee/loved one should ALWAYS wash your hands before and after performing any personal care techniques to prevent the spread of infection.

5. Safety Considerations: Persons with COPD can sometimes experience a "flare up" in their condition. A flare up may also be called an exacerbation. A flare up can be caused by inhaling smoke or other pollutants, a lung infection, a sudden change in weather, too much activity, or stress. Signs of a flare up may include coughing, wheezing, an increase in mucus production, increased anxiety, and/or difficulty sleeping. Signs of a flare up are usually symptoms that last longer and are more intense than usual symptoms that the person experiences. It's best to try to prevent a COPD flare up. Avoid smoke and try to avoid getting an infection. Have hand sanitizer available for the occasions when you and your caregivee/loved one cannot use soap and water. Remain calm and use medications that the doctor has prescribed, as directed. Addressing a flare up early may prevent a hospitalization. If you call the doctor for any reason, always be sure to let the doctor's office know that you are calling about a person who has COPD and let them know if your caregivee/loved one is having difficulty breathing.

Please remember that outside air pollution can impact the person's breathing. Weather can cause an increase in the amount of pollution in the air. Air pollution or respiratory alerts are issued in some geographic locations and on days when there are air pollution alerts, consider staying indoors to reduce their risk of an increase in COPD symptoms.

If your caregivee/loved one is prescribed an antibiotic for an infection, the medication should be taken until it is finished, even if they are feeling better. Only antibiotics prescribed by the physician or other primary care provider, such as a nurse practitioner, should be taken.

If your caregivee/loved one is using oxygen to supplement their COPD treatment plan, the safety guidelines regarding oxygen are extremely important. Oxygen on its own does not explode or burn, but it accelerates what does burn. Any combustible or flammable material and/or any source of ignition such as a match, spark, lighter, or any open flame can quickly cause a serious fire. Oxygen accelerates combustion. Persons who are using oxygen should NEVER smoke while using oxygen and no smoking should be allowed near a person using oxygen. Do not use aerosol sprays near oxygen equipment. "No Smoking" and "Oxygen in Use" signs should be placed where they can be easily seen. Open flames, such as candles or gas stoves, should not be used in a room where oxygen is in use.

Your caregivee/loved one may be using oxygen provided by a "concentrator" that runs on electricity. The company that provides the caregivee/loved one's oxygen should provide you and your caregivee/loved one with "back up" tanks of oxygen in case of a power failure and they should show you how to use them if needed. If they have not done this, ask them to! Demonstrate back to them what you are shown to be certain you are using the equipment safely. Notify the electric power company that your caregivee/loved one is on oxygen; this may help you to receive priority consideration if the power fails. Store oxygen tanks on a flat surface in a well-ventilated room, standing up straight. Turn oxygen off when it is not in use and do not let untrained persons use or adjust oxygen equipment. Do not transport oxygen in the trunk of a car. Ask the doctor, nurse, or other health care team member if you have any questions about your caregivee/loved one and oxygen use.

The company that provides the oxygen equipment may be another resource to use if you have questions about the equipment. Most home medical equipment (HME) or durable medical equipment (DME) companies have respiratory therapists on staff who are experts about oxygen, its delivery, and its use. (These are companies that provide and deliver medical equipment, such as oxygen.) Call the doctor or HME/DME if you have questions. Do not change oxygen settings unless directed to do so by the doctor.

6. When to Call the Doctor, Nurse, or Care Team: These are only possible examples and NOT an inclusive list. Please remember that calling *before* a situation becomes a bigger problem is always best. It's better to catch problems when they are relatively small. It is much harder to address "big" problems.

- Caregivee/loved one is less alert or appears mentally cloudy.
- Caregivee/loved one's lips and nail beds have a bluish tint.
- Caregivee/loved one becomes unusually short of breath when talking.
- Caregivee/loved one is breathing harder and faster than usual. They may be wheezing and the breathing is not made better by the usual methods.
- Caregivee/loved one is experiencing chest pain.
- Caregivee/loved one is feeling unusually tired for no reason, sometimes for days (this may be more common in women).
- Caregivee/loved one experiences lightheadedness or sudden dizziness that is unrelieved by sitting down.
- Caregivee/loved one experiences sudden weight gain of two pounds overnight or five pounds in one week's time.
- Caregivee/loved one experiences any sudden, new symptoms or a change in the pattern of symptoms they already have or if symptoms become stronger or last longer than usual.
- Caregivee/loved one is very emotional, perhaps they cannot stop crying or they are showing other obvious signs of distress. Perhaps they are questioning their spiritual beliefs, or doubting what they once believed.
- Caregivee/loved one has distressful nausea or nausea that won't go away, with or without vomiting.
- Caregivee/loved one has stopped eating or drinking or has difficulty swallowing.
- Caregivee/loved one has a change in how they urinate. Perhaps they cannot urinate or they are urinating much more frequently than usual, but only producing small amounts of urine. Perhaps their urine has changed color, is very dark, and/or has a strong odor.

- Caregivee/loved one has had a change in their bowel movements or has stopped having bowel movements for more than three days, even if they are not eating very much.
- Caregivee/loved one has fallen and is experiencing discomfort after the fall and/or has decreased movement after the fall.
- Caregivee/loved one has a cough that produces dark or blood-tinged sputum. This might also be obvious in their spit/saliva.
- Caregivee/loved one has a higher/faster heart rate than usual that it is unrelieved after resting.
- Caregivee/loved one has unexplained bruising.
- Caregivee/loved one has a sudden or high fever.
- Caregivee/loved one cannot get comfortable/find relief from pain. For example, pain wakes caregivee/loved one up at night or pain comes on suddenly. Always believe whatever your caregivee/loved one tells you about their pain. Caregivee/loved ones are the expert on their pain.
- Caregivee/loved one has white spots or a white coating on their tongue, or any other kind of mouth sore. This may or may not be accompanied by difficulty swallowing.
- Caregivee/loved one has fallen.
- Any other change, complication or concern that you or the caregivee/loved one may have. When in doubt, call!

These are examples only. Your caregivee/loved one might relay to you changes or concerns that vary from those listed here and those concerns should be addressed with your care team.

7. Comfort Considerations: COPD cannot be cured, but there are ways to help a person living with COPD feel more comfortable. The feeling of air movement can provide comfort to a person with breathing difficulties, such as having a fan on. Having the person sit up straight in a chair while leaning forward with their arms or elbows resting on a table in a "tripod" position might facilitate easier breathing.

Persons with advanced COPD may experience "air hunger." Sometimes when this happens it creates anxiety that causes further shortness of breath and the person may feel that they are trapped in a vicious cycle of difficulty breathing and anxiety. Morphine is sometimes prescribed for persons with COPD to slow breathing and address anxiety. Morphine comes in many forms and dosages. It may be prescribed to prevent the feeling of air hunger. It should only be taken as prescribed and please remember that it is always constipating.

If your caregivee/loved one is on any pain medication, they can and, in many cases, do cause constipation. Constipation is a side effect of morphine that does not go away. The doctor may advise taking a stool softener or laxative daily. Morphine may cause nausea and drowsiness in some people, but these side effects often subside after a day or two. Morphine can have a "euphoric" effect in some people and might calm generalized anxiety. Sometimes people fear becoming addicted to morphine. When a drug is used for its intended purpose, it is rarely addicting. A person with advanced COPD has a genuine lack of ability for air exchange. The anxiety associated with not being able to breathe is genuine. Morphine, like oxygen, is best regarded as a comfort measure when prescribed by a doctor for a caregivee/loved one experiencing air hunger. Keep this, and all drugs, out of the reach of children and teenagers.

Comfort for your caregivee /loved one can mean physical, mental, spiritual, or any combination of those kinds of comfort. As a caregiver, providing comfort for your caregivee/ loved one sometimes means "the small things." Small things are sometimes easily overlooked. Having regular bowel movements may seem like a small thing, but it is actually a very large part of comfort. If your caregivee/loved one is on any pain medication, or if they use morphine or a morphine type drug to address symptoms of air hunger, it can, and very likely will, cause constipation. Unfortunately, the health care team may sometimes forget to tell you this! It is always better to prevent a problem than to correct a problem, and this is never more true than when it comes to pain medications and constipation. We encourage you not to be shy about asking your caregivee/loved one about their bowel habits and call the doctor or clinic if their bowels have not moved for three days. This is true even if they are not eating very much.

Sometimes distraction, such as watching TV or a movie, reading, or playing cards is enough to ease a person's anxiety. Spending time with a beloved pet is often wonderful therapy for those who are feeling emotionally "down" or depressed. If your caregivee/loved one is spiritually inclined, a visit to their place of worship or from a clergy member may be helpful. A visit to a place that is spiritually meaningful may be comforting. As always, ask your caregivee/loved one since they are the best person to guide you in what they need. Also consider meditation for comfort, especially meditation that focuses on deep breathing.

Your caregivee/loved one may experience difficulty sleeping at night. They may experience shortness of breath and/or coughing when they lie flat. Naps during the daytime may help if the person is feeling tired from lack of sleep. Using more than one pillow to prop the head and upper body up may help. Keeping the head and chest elevated by raising the mattress from underneath is often comforting. The doctor, nurse, or health care team may suggest the caregivee/loved one purchase a foam "wedge" to lay on or to position under the mattress to facilitate breathing. A reclining chair or hospital bed can also be considered.

Sometimes your caregivee/loved one may ask to be left alone for awhile. Please don't take this personally! Living with a respiratory illness disrupts a person's whole life, and it affects those around them, including, and perhaps especially, the caregiver. Give your caregivee/loved one time to "regroup" if they ask for it, and use this time to do something nice for yourself. If your caregivee/loved one doesn't recover from their need to be alone after a day or two, it's time to talk to them about it, and, very possibly, it's time to call the doctor, nurse, or other health care team member.

A person may experience dry mouth when on certain respiratory medicines, especially if they use oxygen therapy and/or inhalers. Sucking on ice chips or hard candy can relieve dry mouth. Maintaining a clean, fresh mouth is a comfort measure. Attentive mouth care may prevent and help detect mouth problems at an early stage. Persons with COPD often have a weakened immune system, and some medications, such as inhalers and steroids, can put the person at risk for mouth infections. Notify the doctor, nurse, or health care team if your caregivee/loved one develops any mouth sores or a white coating on their tongue. Rinse after using inhalers if directed to do so.

Persons with COPD often feel anxious, depressed, and sometimes grouchy. They may feel fearful performing daily tasks that were once routine and they may be grieving their ability to breathe normally. Allow them to go at their own pace as much as possible. Try to be an "active listener." An active listener listens to the person's fears and experiences without interrupting. Patience on the caregiver's part might be appreciated because a person with COPD may need to speak slowly to accommodate their breathing. Allow the person to draw their own conclusions, and, for some people, verbalizing feelings provides great relief. Your caregivee/loved one may express a range of emotions as they adjust to their circumstances. Help your caregivee/loved one to avoid stressful situations and stressful people. If your caregivee/loved one is having difficulty sleeping at night and/or if they have anxiety that is not well addressed with non-pharmaceutical measures, have them speak with their doctor. An anti-anxiety medication may be in order.

8. Special Considerations: Unfortunately, the stress that COPD causes on the body will eventually take its toll. Sometimes, as a person approaches the end of life, the caregivee/loved one, the doctor, and the caregiver may wish to consider either palliative care or hospice care. For more information and resources related to these types of care please refer to the section entitled "End-of-Life, Palliative, and Hospice Care."

9. Special Instructions Given to You by the Doctor, Nurse, or Care Team:

_____

_____

_____

_____

_____

_____

_____

_____

_____

10. Resources:

- The American Academy of Allergy Asthma & Immunology offers an explanation of the differences between asthma and COPD: http://www.aaaai.org/conditions-and-treatments/library/asthma-library/asthma-and-copd-differences-and-similarities.aspx
- MedlinePlus offers a COPD section explaining the disease and common symptoms: http://www.nlm.nih.gov/medlineplus/copd.html
- The Centers for Disease Control and Prevention offers a What is COPD? Resource: http://www.cdc.gov/copd/
- The National Heart, Lung, and Blood Institute also offers a What is COPD resource including treatment and living with the disease sections: http://www.nhlbi.nih.gov/health/health-topics/topics/copd
- The National Heart, Lung, and Blood Institute offers a What Are the Lungs? page as well for more information

on how this organ is affected: http://www.nhlbi.nih.gov/
health/health-topics/topics/hlw/

- NIH Senior Health has information about treating COPD:
  http://nihseniorhealth.gov/copd/treatingcopd/01.html
- The COPD Foundation has a frequently asked questions
  page for caregivers: http://www.copdfoundation.org/Learn-
  More/For-Patients-Caregivers/FAQ-for-Caregivers.aspx

References

Ford, ES, Croft, JB, Mannino, DM, Wheaton, AG, Zhang, X, Giles, WH.
(2013). COPD surveillance-United States, 1999–2011. *Chest Journal*,
144(1): 284–305. doi: 10.1378/chest.13-0809.

DIABETES CARE

1. Introduction: Diabetes, also known as Diabetes Mellitus (DM), is a disorder caused by not enough insulin being produced by the body or by the body being unable to use the insulin that it produces. Insulin is very important because it helps the body to sort and utilize carbohydrates and sugars from the foods we eat. Diabetes is usually a lifelong illness. Children as well as adults can have diabetes. Treatment includes diet and exercise, and oral medication or insulin injections are often part of the treatment for diabetes as well. Unfortunately, diabetes is the most common cause of blindness, kidney failure, and amputations in adults. Research provided by the Centers for Disease Control and Prevention (CDC) reports that as of June, 2014, 29.1 million people in the United States were diagnosed as having diabetes (CDC, 2014). In 2012, 1.7 million people were 20 years of age or older when they were diagnosed (CDC, 2014). For more information about diabetes visit: http://www.cdc.gov/diabetes. You will find more diabetes-specific resources listed at the end of this chapter.

You may refer to other chapters in this book such as: "Amputation Care," "Cardiac Care," "Stroke Care (Cerebrovascular Accident)," and "Bedbound Care (Care of the Immobilized or Bedridden Patient)."

2. General Information: Persons who take insulin must eat a certain amount of calories each day, as directed by their doctor or diabetes educator. Depending upon the type of diabetes your caregivee/loved one has, they may be required to have healthy snacks in the afternoon or at bedtime. Persons living with diabetes do best if they establish and follow a routine of eating at specific times during the day. They may have life-threatening problems if they are unable, or if they choose not to, eat as required. The good news is that diabetes can be controlled and the long-term, negative effects of diabetes are decreased when the person follows the recommended lifestyle changes.

Circulation, which means how the blood flows through the body, may be affected in persons with diabetes. As these changes occur, people may "lose feeling" or have decreased sensation in their hands and feet. Some people with diabetes have pain or a burning sensation in their extremities when their circulation is affected. This pain is called "neuropathy." Sadly, these circulatory problems may result in amputations of a toe or a lower extremity. Other complications of diabetes can include poor eyesight or blindness, the development of vascular skin ulcers, kidney problems, heart problems, and stroke.

Your caregivee/loved one may have met with a "diabetes educator" as they learned about their illness. These diabetes educators, also called certified diabetes educators (CDEs) are usually RNs or dietitians and they are a good source of information regarding this complex illness. We encourage you to work with them closely.

3. General Goals for Care: Bottom line goal: establish a routine that follows the advice of your doctor, nurse, diabetes educator, or other health care team members and stick to it. Establishing a routine in diabetes management will keep your caregivee/loved one safe *and* comfortable and may help prevent the complications associated with diabetes or keep them from worsening. Your caregivee/loved one's routine will involve nutritious meals, served at the same time every day, and possibly medication or insulin, also taken at the same time every day, again, as directed.

A person with diabetes may be instructed to check blood sugars daily, or more frequently, and this should become part of the routine as well, done at the same time(s) every day. The blood sugar numbers/results should be written down as part of the daily routine. The doctor, nurse, or health care team uses the person's blood sugar numbers to make adjustments to the diet, medication, and/or insulin. It's a good idea to keep a log of these blood sugar numbers, using a small note-book or a calendar. You and your caregivee/loved one will refer to this log often. In fact, when checking glucose levels, it is important to note that sometimes change in glucose values can be an early sign of infection in caregivee/loved ones with diabetes. And the doctor, nurse, or health care team may want to see these blood sugar numbers as they were recorded over time (several days in a row). Being able to provide these numbers can help prevent emergencies and may prevent an emergency room visit. Call the doctor right away if there is an unusually high or low number. The health care team will tell you what "unusually" high or low numbers are for your caregivee/loved one.

Diabetes doesn't "go away." It is always "running in the background" of the person's life and, because of this, it might be easy for you or your caregivee/loved one to forget that diabetes needs to be addressed during changes that may be seen as "routine." Changes may need to be made to the person's daily regimen if they have a cold or influenza (flu) for example. The doctor, nurse, or other team member might make small but important changes to your caregivee/loved one's routine, perhaps making medication changes, and it is important to follow these recommendations.

A person with diabetes may lose sensation in their extremities or have vision problems. Older adults may be at an increased risk to trip or fall. For more information, refer to Chapter Six: Safety in the Home: The Most Frequent Health Care Setting of Choice! A fall can cause a wound, and caregivee/loved ones with diabetes may not "feel" the same sensations and may have a skin tear or wound from falling or tripping. If your caregivee/loved one develops a wound of any kind let the doctor know right away. Keeping your caregivee/loved one's skin clean and dry, especially their feet, is very important. What your caregivee/loved one wears every day is another part of the daily routine and we address this more in the next section.

4. Personal Care Considerations: Persons with diabetes have poor circulation and decreased sensation in their hands and feet, so they may be unable to tell how warm their bath/shower temperature is. It is very important to always check the temperature of the water before your caregivee/loved one gets in the tub or shower. Foot care is a very important part of your caregivee/loved one's routine—inspect the feet and keep the feet clean and dry. DO NOT CUT YOUR CAREGIVEE/LOVED ONE'S TOENAILS. Usually a podiatrist or their doctor, not a nail technician, should cut their toenails. Doing this may lead to a very bad wound. Usually a podiatrist or other specialist cuts the nails of persons with diabetes. It is a good idea to dry between the toes after a bath or shower, and this is a good time to inspect the skin for any types of break in the skin. Make this part of the daily routine. Even a small wound in a person with diabetes can become a big problem. If you see a break in the skin or any other skin change, let your doctor, nurse, or health care team know about it right away. Ask a member of the care team if lotion applied to the skin and if foot rubs are a good idea. Doing this may increase blood flow and keep the skin supple.

Your caregivee/loved one *should never walk with bare feet.* What your caregivee/loved one wears on their feet is very important. They should wear clean, dry socks that are not too big or small, and socks with tight elastic bands at the tops should be avoided. Pharmacies or pharmaceutical stores sell socks for people with diabetes. Properly fitted shoes are important for a person with diabetes. Toes and feet should always be protected in shoes that are not too big or too small. And slippers should not have elastic in them which could be tight and interfere with blood flow. Any restriction in blood flow may cause a skin problem for your caregivee/loved one. Be mindful of swelling. If your caregivee/loved one's feet swell, their shoes may be tight. This might cause rubbing and lead to a pressured area which could quickly become a wound.

5. Safety Considerations: It is important to keep your caregivee/loved one's living areas neat and free of any objects that could be stepped on or tripped over. Pathways should be kept clear and lighting bright enough so that those with decreased vision can move about safely.

The doctor, nurse, or other health care team member will

have told you and your caregivee/loved one what a "normal" or "healthy" blood sugar number should be. If a blood sugar reading drops too low or goes too high a person with diabetes may act differently than usual. This requires *immediate attention*. Contact a health care team member and ask for instructions. When you call, be sure to tell them you are calling about a person with diabetes who has an either high or low blood sugar number. Sometimes a person with low blood sugar has experienced this before and may ask you for some orange juice, which can be used to treat low blood sugar right away while you call the health care team for further instructions. The symptoms of low or high blood sugar are very serious and can "look" different in various people. Call the doctor, nurse, or other health care team with any questions.

6. When to Call the Doctor, Nurse, or Care Team: These are only possible examples and NOT an inclusive list. Please remember that calling *before* a situation becomes a bigger problem is always best. It's better to catch problems when they are relatively small. It is much harder to address "big" problems.

- Caregivee/loved one shows symptoms of low blood sugar: perspiration (sweating), feeling hungry, feeling weak, feeling light headed, tremors (shaky hands/arms), acting anxious or nervous, nausea, complaints of nightmares, restless sleep, confusion.
- Caregivee/loved one shows symptoms of high blood sugar: thirst, breath smells "fruity," increased urination, abdominal ("belly") pain, nausea, weakness, lethargy (slow movements, unsure of their movements), weight loss.

- Caregivee/loved one develops a wound of any kind, but especially on the feet or lower legs.
- Caregivee/loved one has a change in how they urinate. Perhaps they cannot urinate or they are urinating much more frequently than usual but only producing small amounts of urine. Perhaps their urine has changed color, is very dark, and/or has a strong odor.
- Caregivee/loved one shows signs and symptoms of a cold or influenza (flu).
- Caregivee/loved one has a sudden or high fever.
- Caregivee/loved one has had a change in their bowel movements or has stopped having bowel movements for more than three days.
- Caregivee/loved one starts a new medication that the diabetes health care team does not know about. This includes vitamins and any over-the-counter medications such as a cough syrup or laxative.
- Caregivee/loved one is not eating or is eating foods high in sugar.
- Caregivee/loved one has fallen.
- Caregivee/loved one has a wound that is not healing.

These are examples only. Your caregivee/loved one might relay to you changes or concerns that vary from those listed here and those concerns should be addressed with your care team.

7. Comfort Considerations: Comfort for your caregivee/loved one can mean physical, mental, spiritual, or any combination of those kinds of comfort. As a caregiver, providing comfort for your caregivee/loved one sometimes means "the small things." Small things are sometimes easily overlooked. Having regular bowel movements may seem like a small thing, but it is actually a very large part of comfort. If your caregivee/loved one is on any pain medication, they can and, in many cases, do cause constipation. Call a health team member if your caregivee/loved one has not had a bowel movement for three days. You will be guided toward treatment that will be best for a person with diabetes; that is, one that will not affect their blood sugar levels.

In regards to physical discomfort, changing positions or a gentle back rub and/or massage may help. A heating pad and/or cold/ice compress should *not* be used on those with diabetes unless directed by the doctor, nurse, or health team member. These items can be dangerous to a caregivee/loved one with diabetes.

8. Special Considerations: It is always better to address any potential problems or concerns earlier rather than later, and this is perhaps more true with diabetes than with any other illness, especially in regards to wounds. The diabetes educator may be able to guide you to local services, such as diabetes education programs, foot clinics/programs, and support/meeting groups for caregivee/loved ones with diabetes and/or their caregivers in your area.

9. Special Instructions Given to You by the Doctor, Nurse, or Care Team:

_____

_____

_____

_____

_____

_____

_____

_____

_____

10. Resources:

- Many diabetes resources are offered from the National Diabetes Education Program: http://ndep.nih.gov/
- These include Guiding Principles for the Care of People With or at Risk for Diabetes and I Have Diabetes: http://ndep.nih.gov/hcp-businesses-and-schools/guiding-principles/
http://ndep.nih.gov/i-have-diabetes/
- The Centers for Disease Control and Preventions provide resources including the basics of the disease and treatment options: http://www.cdc.gov/diabetes/basics/index.html
- 8 Tips for Caregivers for those caregiving for diabetes from the American Diabetes Association: http://www.diabetes.org/living-with-diabetes/recently-diagnosed/8-tips-for-caregivers.html
- Diabetes: Treating Wounds and Injuries from WedMD: http://www.webmd.com/a-to-z-guides/wound-care-10/diabetic-wounds
- Tips for Diabetes Caregivers from the Mayo Clinic: http://www.mayoclinic.org/diseases-conditions/diabetes/expert-blog/diabetes-caregiver/bgp-20056489
- The Health Resources and Services Administration offers information about amputation through their Lower

Extremity Amputation Prevention (LEAP) program's site: http://www.hrsa.gov/hansensdisease/leap/

Reference

Centers for Disease Control and Prevention (CDC). (2014). National Diabetes Statistics Report, 2014. Retrieved from http://www.cdc.gov/diabetes/pubs/statsreport14/national-diabetes-report-web.pdf

END-OF-LIFE, PALLIATIVE, AND HOSPICE CARE

1. Introduction: As the population ages, it goes without saying that we all have a limited time on this earth. Trying to make each day the best it can be must be a goal for both care-givers and their caregivee/loved ones. Just by watching TV, it is easy to see that we live in a death-denying and death-defying culture. People on TV come back to life full of health after "dying" and experiencing CPR (cardiopulmonary resuscitation). Rescue medicine can "save" anyone. The fact is we will all die and so having input about our wishes and experiences is a very good and important thing. Knowing what we and loved ones want can bring enormous comfort to those we love and care for. There are projects about how to have "the conversation" because people have difficulty or discomfort talking about anything related to the end of life. The time to have that conversation is not in the emergency department or an intensive care unit with strangers—sadly, this is a rushed, chaotic, and somewhat impersonal setting and no matter how nice or how kind they may be, they do not truly "know" you and your caregivee/loved one. It should not be a dialogue that is a "one time and done" conversation by any means; this should be an ongoing conversation. Numerous studies report that people prefer to die at home, and in the past ten years, an increasing number of Americans died at home rather than in the hospital (Centers for Disease Control and Prevention [CDC], 2013). Even so, nearly 50% of all Americans still die in a hospital and almost 70% die in a hospital, nursing home, or long-term-care facility (PBS, 2010). This is despite the fact that 70% of Americans report that they would prefer to die at home (PBS, 2010). Amongst Americans with chronic diseases, this number is even higher: 80% of these caregivee/loved ones prefer not to be in the hospital or in intensive care when they are dying (PBS, 2010).

Having been very privileged to be a registered nurse and knowing what the best hospice care is or "looks like," I am a proponent. At the same time, because so many people no longer die at home, but in other settings such as a hospital, we no longer see death integrated into our daily life. In the "olden" days, in the best scenarios, people got sick and were cared for by a loved one, then died at home, surrounded by those they cared about and who cared about them—perhaps more importantly. Either way, before Medicare reimbursement was initiated in 1966, people generally stayed home and death was "attended" by family and friends.

This goal of making each day the best it can be, sometimes in very difficult circumstances and with varying health problems, should be the goal for care of all people, whether or not they are at the end of life. And perhaps it should take place at home. The fact that we should treat all caregivee/ loved ones like we treat hospice caregivee/loved ones dawned on me after knowing "enough to know" about hospice; by that I mean after learning enough about it to understand it and ask questions about it. Concepts like being comfortable and being educated to the fact that sometimes it is necessary and okay to take strong medications for pain, that symptom management often needs to include medications for anxiety, and that, perhaps, it's time for people to not be afraid to discuss spiritual pain and to be able to incorporate spiritual aspects of care into all care. We should try to eliminate or decrease suffering and discomfort whenever possible. A favorite meal prepared and brought to the home by a long-time friend is just one example of the best part, a meaningful part, of care in the home.

We need to work toward accepting that death is inevitable and that palliative and end-of-life (EOL) care, for example, hospice care at home, is one way to sometimes more compassionately and effectively manage symptoms. To be cared for and spend time with friends and family (rather than be in an impersonal setting with strangers) in a setting that may be cherished and more comfortable is often the wish at the end of life. There are instances where hospice is also provided in a hospital, skilled nursing, or nursing facility based on the person's unique needs. In this way, they also get the best components of caring at the end of life regardless of the setting.

Let's take a moment to consider why one might be more comfortable at home. At the hospital, there are usually visiting hours and age limits on visitors. Grandchildren might not be able to visit, for example. In most hospitals, the caregivee/loved one wears a gown like all the other caregivee/loved ones (and no matter what anyone says—they are still ugly!). Meal time and food choices are often limited and/or scheduled for ease of preparation and delivery to a volume of caregivee/loved ones. There are other parameters as well that must exist when services are provided in a large building designed to care for a lot of people. Put another way, a hospital is not a restful, quiet environment to hold sacred conversations and address end-of-life care issues. Now—think of your favorite "home" place. There are no visiting hours and no age limits on the visitors. You are in charge of your kitchen, your refrigerator's contents, and meal times. Your pets, who you might consider to be part of your family and who may be a great source of comfort, can be around you. You can play your favorite music or TV shows at whatever volume you like. There are numerous other comfort considerations that make home a much more desirable setting! The contents of this chapter are appropriate for most persons at the end of life, not only those who chose hospice services. The compassionate care and other information has applicability for most people in that stage of life.

Please refer to the other sections of this book for guidance of your caregivee/loved one's specific care considerations. Some chapters might include: "Cancer Care" and "Bedbound Care (Care of the Immobilized or Bedridden Patient)."

2. General Information: Hospice is not driven by a specific diagnosis; it is usually appropriate when a person has an average life expectancy of six months or less if the illness runs a natural course. There may not be one single diagnosis, but many diagnoses that combined make hospice care the appropriate choice. It all depends upon the individual person's complex status. In fact, most people do not have just one health care problem. For example, a person may have a chronic (long-term) illness, such as cancer, diabetes, heart failure, hypertension, Alzheimer's disease or dementia, and/or other health care problems. This is particularly true for older adults.

Much care is directed toward people at the end of life. There are different models of end-of-life care and palliative care is one model. The goal of palliative care is to make a person feel better whether or not they are still receiving curative treatment (MedlinePlus, n.d.). Hospice care is also one of those special services and is a type of palliative care. Hospice care is often chosen when curative measures are no longer effective or the burden of that care is too difficult for a person to continue. For some people and families, there comes a time when they wish to stop invasive or more aggressive treatment. In fact, hospice team members are especially skilled in providing information and having difficult conversations when this time comes. A hospice nurse can visit a caregivee/loved one at any time to evaluate their appropriateness for hospice services. Hospice care services are often provided in a home care setting, but the person can be evaluated and cared for in any care setting.

Hospice is a philosophy of care that recognizes that death is a part of living. This means that when hospice care is chosen, this philosophy follows the person and caregiver across caregivee/loved one care settings. Hospice care can be delivered in the home, in the hospital, in nursing facilities, and assisted living facilities, but most hospice care is provided in the home (American Cancer Society, 2014). This is because it has been shown that most people prefer to be at home in familiar surroundings at the end of life.

Hospice in the home means that a team of professionals, called an "interdisciplinary team," will visit you and your caregivee/loved one at regular intervals at your home. If you've been providing care for your caregivee/loved one in the home, you will be a valuable asset to the hospice team because you will know your loved one's unique needs. Hospice services are usually provided by a local visiting nurse agency (VNA) or a hospice organization. Contact your local VNA or hospice if you have any questions relating to their specific admission criteria for hospice services.

When the hospice team visits you and your caregivee/ loved one, the team will be administering care and teaching you, as the caregiver, how to provide the best care to your loved one. One of the best things about hospice is that care is directed toward the caregivee/loved one *and* family. You, as the caregiver, are embraced and also cared for in this unique care model.

Your hospice team may consist of: a hospice physician and/or your caregivee/loved one's primary care physician (PCP), a hospice nurse, home health aides or hospice aides, a social worker, a chaplain (sometimes called a spiritual care coordinator), and hospice trained volunteers. Sometimes, other professionals join the team for short periods of time to address your caregivee/loved one's particular needs. These "allied professionals" might include a physical therapist or an occupational therapist. Hospice care is most often paid for by Medicare, Medicaid, VA, or private insurance.

There are also specialized bereavement counselors to support you, the caregiver, and/or family members or the caregivee/loved one's spouse after the death of your caregivee/ loved one. For Medicare, bereavement services may follow you and your family for up to a year, depending on a number of factors.

And don't worry: The whole team does not show up on your doorstep at one time. Visits are planned according to you and your caregivee/loved one's needs. When/if needs increase, the visits may increase. If your caregivee/loved one's status is very stable, you may see your hospice team members less often. The Medicare hospice benefit provides four levels of care. These different levels of care are available when/if they are needed to manage your caregivee/loved one's symptoms. Your caregivee/loved one can move from one level of care and back as needed to manage pain and symptoms.

Continuous Care: If your caregivee/loved one has uncontrolled pain or symptoms, continuous care may be appropriate. This level of care is provided in the person's residence where nursing and other hospice care can be provided continuously, for hours or days, until the symptoms are managed and the crisis passes. Once symptoms are under control, care changes back to the Routine Home Care level.

General Inpatient Care: If your caregivee/loved one has symptoms that cannot reasonably be managed in the home, inpatient care may be available. This way the caregivee/loved one can be monitored closely and treatments and medications can be adjusted until the caregivee/loved one is comfortable. Once symptoms are under control, the caregivee/loved one will return home.

Routine Home Care: This is the most common level of care and includes regular visits by the hospice interdisciplinary team to the residence. This level of care is for persons who have well-controlled symptoms and can remain comfortably in their home. Most hospice care is provided at this level.

Respite Care: Providing care around the clock is often exhausting and stressful. It is important that caregivers take care of themselves as well. Respite is a short-term (five consecutive days) level of care designed to provide the caregiver with a "respite" from caregiving responsibilities. This respite may be to relax, attend to personal healthcare needs, visit family, attend a function, or for other needs.

The following is an illustration of what hospice care might "look" like when it is delivered in the home, and how a hospice team "works" when delivering care in the home. The hospice team, under the guidance of the hospice physician and usually in conjunction with your caregivee/loved one's primary care physician, will provide care, but, perhaps more importantly, they will also teach you how to care for your caregivee/loved one in the home as they move toward the end of life. The hospice physician may also make home visits. Your caregivee/loved one's hospice nurse will likely be the "care manager" or "case manager" and will coordinate your caregivee/loved one's plan for care and home visits with you, your caregivee/loved one, and the various other hospice team members. This plan includes visit frequency, medications, medical equipment, and other services.

The hospice interdisciplinary team meets regularly and discusses your caregivee/loved one's particular care needs in depth. Again, hospice focuses on the family, not just the person receiving care. Of course the person is the "jewel in the crown," but hospice appreciates that as the caregiver, you may have questions and concerns, perhaps about the increased care needs or about grief once they pass away. And the hospice team is there to support you, as well as the caregivee/loved one. If there are other family members or friends who are also participating in the care, they are supported as well.

By the time hospice care is initiated, life may seem to have become hectic to both the caregiver and caregivee/loved one. Especially in the first few days or weeks of hospice care, days can be busy and, as the caregiver, you may feel a bit over-whelmed as many pieces of the end-of-life puzzle are put into place. You may notice a "shift" in the focus of care. Prior to hospice care, the care team was doing all they could, some-times very aggressively and with lots of doctor visits and other appointments and treatments, to cure them. Now, you will see the hospice team calmly and quietly addressing the pain and symptoms rather than trying to cure the illness or cause of the pain. You may see care being provided in the home that you wished you could have had long before! Hospice care is very comprehensive, meaning far reaching and very inclu-sive. The care team looks not only at the person's symptoms and caregiver(s), but also at the "whole" caregivee/loved one. Care is provided to address physical, mental, and spiritual well-being.

The hospice team, in large part, is present in your home to teach and support you and your caregivee/loved one. Because of time, staffing, and financial constraints, the hospice team cannot provide care in your home 24 hours a day, but they are "on call" to answer your questions 24 hours a day. The hospice social worker may be able to provide you with infor-mation about other in-home services should they be needed.

At every visit, the hospice nurse, usually a registered nurse (RN), often a nurse specially certified in end-of-life care, will assess the caregivee/loved one; see how you, the primary caregiver, are doing; and assess how other family members are doing as well. The nurse cannot provide medical or nursing care for caregivers and family members, of course, but they will be supportive and informative and will make recommen-dations to the hospice team as needed.

As an example, perhaps you, the caregiver, need a break to

keep a doctor's appointment for yourself, but you have no one to stay with your caregivee/loved one. The hospice nurse may recommend to the team that a volunteer is needed to stay with your caregivee/loved one for an hour or two while you attend your appointment. In this scenario, you will then hear from the volunteer coordinator. The volunteer coordinator will speak with you and your caregivee/loved one to match a hospice-trained volunteer to meet your family's particular care needs. In a perfect world, the caregivee/loved one and the volunteer have something in common, like a hobby, or have had military service. Because the volunteer has been trained to work with people who are near their end of life, they will know that it is most acceptable in certain cases to just sit quietly and be a presence if that is all that is needed and/or family wishes. Feel free to discuss your desires with the volunteer coordinator ahead of time to help them match the right volunteer to you and your caregivee/loved one. Hospice volunteers are often referred to as "the Heart of Hospice." According to the National Hospice and Palliative Care Organization (NHPCO) there are 355,000 hospice volunteers in the U.S. and in 2013 they provided 16 million hours of service (NHPCO, 2014).

The hospice team is also responsible for delivery of medical equipment that may be needed for the caregivee/loved one's comfort and safety. This equipment might include a hospital bed, a bedside commode, a shower bench, or other equipment. As your caregivee/loved one's needs change, the hospice care team will help decide what equipment best meets those needs. As the illness progresses, you and/or the caregivee/loved one may be feeling more emotional and hardly have time to feel or process these emotions because, as your caregivee/loved one's health declines, their care needs increase. The hospice team will hopefully have guided you down the path that you find yourself on. Yes, it is difficult. It is perhaps your first time dealing with a person who is nearing their end of life. Find solace in the fact that your hospice team is made up of professionals who chose end-of-life care as their vocation. They may be the nicest, most consistent, reliable, and caring team that you have yet to meet in any care setting. We hope that this is your experience.

Your hospice nurse will have been ahead of the process, preparing you for changes and the possible realization that soon your loved one may no longer be able to get out of bed. Perhaps you were seeing it with your own eyes, but still needed a trusted member of the hospice team to tell you what you were seeing to realize what was happening. This is okay, and a part of the process.

The hospice team will help prepare you for the physical, mental, and emotional challenges that may lie ahead. They listen to the concerns that you and your caregivee/loved one may have, and, as needed, and only with consent of the person and caregiver(s), they can refer other hospice team members to help guide you. It is important to note that team members visit only if this is the desire of the person and family. Some persons like to meet all of the interdisciplinary hospice team members while other persons and families prefer to see the hospice nurse and/or the hospice aide or other team members only. Expect the hospice nurse to make recommendations about team support according to needs that they identify for your caregivee/loved one and based on their experience.

The hospice nurse teaches, often by demonstration, how

to provide specific physical care of your caregivee/loved one, tailored to their particular needs. For example, the nurse may show you how to turn your caregivee/loved one in bed and how to administer medication that might be needed to address their symptoms. The hospice nurse may see that you need help providing personal care for your caregivee/loved one and, if this is the case, they may direct hospice aides to come to the house and provide a bed bath one or more days a week. If the nurse sees that you or your caregivee/loved one need support, they listen, assess, and make the appropriate recommendations.

The hospice nurse, after discussion with the caregivee/loved one, may recommend that the hospice chaplain, sometimes called the "spiritual care coordinator," make a home visit if they appear to be experiencing a time of spiritual questioning. The hospice nurse is in regular contact with the hospice physician (or the caregivee/loved one's PCP) to discuss the physical and emotional well-being of your caregivee/loved one. Medications may be added or adjusted to address symptoms, such as pain or anxiety. Some other medications may be discontinued. Your hospice nurse will review with you why this is done. And if they do not, ask!

Hopefully, through this illustration, you can see how the hospice team works together to provide the particular and individualized care that will best meet your caregivee/loved one's unique needs. There is planned communication and co-ordination with collaborations between and among members of the entire team.

3. General Goals for Care: Bottom line goal: Comfort. Hospice philosophy encourages non-aggressive and non-invasive measures that are gently applied to help the person and caregiver feel better and more comfortable. These measures are provided with tender loving care. The care embodies respect and dignity for a caregivee/loved one as they near the end of life. This care is to help the person have a symptom-controlled and dignified death.

When a person is referred to hospice care, usually they have had a discussion with their physician(s) and a mutual decision has been made to stop aggressive treatment, and to only manage symptoms. They have decided to let nature "take its course." Quantity of life is less the focus of their treatment plan and quality of life becomes the true focus of their treatment plan. It does NOT mean that medical treatment is withdrawn. It means that the focus of care for your caregivee/loved one has moved from a "cure" model to a "care" model. This means making every day the best it can be.

What does effective symptom management "look like?" Life becomes calmer. There is less of the "hurry up and wait" experience often associated with appointments at physicians' offices and in other health care settings such as "the lab" (laboratory) and/or the "ED" (emergency department). There may be no more or far fewer "needle sticks" because these can often be painful and are considered "invasive." There may be fewer trips to the pharmacy. There may be less overall worry because a decision has been made to accept that dying is a part of living. The person may feel a sense of calm as they receive this inevitable truth and integrate it into their thoughts. Many express feeling a sense of relief. Perhaps not surprisingly, persons who accept a symptom-management or a "comfort-measures-only" care plan often have a better quality of life and some even live longer than those who accept aggressive treatment right up to the end of life (Temel, et al., 2010).

Sometimes, the caregiver might not agree at all! Or, the caregiver might experience the same sense of relief. Often, the caregivee/loved one accepts the knowledge that they are dying before the caregiver does. The caregiver may be disappointed that the caregivee/loved one, in their view, has "given up" the search for a cure. The caregiver, if they have been providing care for awhile, may experience a feeling of "let down." Perhaps even a feeling of "all that work for no good end." But they may also feel relief. Perhaps they have not been able to express openly how difficult of a task caregiving can be, or that they knew in their heart of hearts that it was unlikely the caregivee/loved one would survive their illness, and were so sad to see them suffer. And it *is* hard to see those we love suffer through treatment after treatment. Perhaps the caregiver sees light at the end of the tunnel and maybe they even feel guilty for having these thoughts. The hospice team anticipates caregivers will experience a myriad of these and other feelings. And they are there to help not only the person receiving care, but you as the caregiver as well.

This is the beauty of hospice care: it is family-focused and the caregiver means as much to the hospice team as the person does. They are there to support you through the process. By the time a person has said "yes" to hospice care, they have usually long since settled their feelings about being near the end of life. The person is often "the first to know" that they are dying, that treatments have stopped working. And sometimes, they are very relieved that the family now also understands this too. It may have been a decision that they delayed making because they did not want to hurt their loved ones' feelings. In many families and cultures, death is simply not talked about. It is not considered a "nice" or socially appropriate topic. A great sigh of relief often enters the caregivee/loved one–caregiver relationship when the decision to choose hospice care has been made.

Let's talk about medications. And to do that effectively, we will be talking about "symptoms" at the same time. And we cannot talk about either of those things without explaining a bit more about how hospice "works." Like the body, many systems are interwoven. Rest assured that your hospice team knows these "interwoven workings," and a large part of the hospice team's job is to help you navigate through them.

Medications that the doctor might stop are those medications that are prescribed in an effort to cure the illness that is threatening the person's life. For example, if Mr. B. has lung cancer *and* high blood pressure and chooses to receive hospice care because his physician told him that his lung cancer cannot be cured, Mr. B. may be told to stop taking chemotherapy medication. Chemotherapy medication is an attempt to cure cancer, in most cases. But Mr. B. would usually (it all depends on the person and the doctor) be instructed to continue to take his high blood pressure medication. Similarly, if Mr. B., still receiving hospice, develops a urinary tract infection (UTI), he may receive antibiotics to treat the infection and prevent unwanted symptoms.

Again, it seems important to stress that under hospice care *medical treatment is not withheld.* If Medicare is paying for the hospice care, hospice will cover medications related to pain and symptom management. Other medicines not related to the terminal illness will continue to be covered however they were covered before hospice care began.

The hospice physician and/or the person's PCP will order medication to keep your caregivee/loved one comfortable. Most persons experience some symptoms at the end-of-life, such as pain, nausea, anxiety, or depression. And the hospice team's expertise lies in this important symptom management. Always report any symptoms and allow them to guide you if your caregivee/loved one develops any new symptoms or if any of their symptoms worsen. The person may have difficulty sleeping and, depending upon their disease, they may have difficulty breathing. Experiencing these symptoms impacts quality of life. They may seem like small things, but they are not.

When a person has only months to live, hospice's approach is to keep them comfortable according to how they define comfort. As an example, you may see the hospice nurse ask your caregivee/loved one to rate their pain on a scale of 1 to 10, with 1 being the least pain and 10 being very bad, or the worst pain. Your caregivee/loved one may report the pain being a "6" on that 1 to 10 scale. But they may be comfortable at that level and not wish to take pain medication because they prefer not to feel "groggy" or tired. Another person may say that they have pain that is a "2," find it intolerable, and request pain medication. The person is always considered the "expert" regarding their own pain level, and their personal tolerance to pain should be respected. Always believe your caregivee/loved one when they tell you that they are in pain! The hospice nurse will educate about the pain medication when/if it is prescribed.

People sometimes fear becoming "addicted" to pain medication. Pain medication, if used for the purpose that it was prescribed for, is very rarely addicting. The person may also have increased pain or develop what is known as "tolerance" to pain medication and the dose may need to be adjusted over time. Because the medication is being prescribed for pain and the goal is always comfort, it is reasonable to anticipate that the medication dosage may be increased, by the physician, if needed.

In hospice care, the doctor may prescribe medication that might be adjusted as needed, within certain parameters. This is called a "range" and is done as a convenience for the caregiver and their caregivee/loved one so that if they experience more pain unexpectedly on a weekend or during the night, the dose may be increased to address pain. In this way, your caregivee/loved one does not have to spend time in pain waiting for you to call the hospice nurse and for the hospice nurse to call back.

The goal of hospice is to maximize the quality of the time that a person has left on this earth. The hospice nurse will guide you. Never increase your caregivee/loved one's pain medication or any other medications if the hospice nurse or doctor has not told you to do so. Hospice medications should only be administered as ordered and if you have any questions, contact the nurse, doctor, or the hospice team.

As your caregivee/loved one moves into their final days, care needs increase and they will very likely become bedbound. You will be taught the care of a bedbound caregivee/loved one. This may include how to give a bed bath, how to turn them, and how to provide other comfort measures, such as using pillows to help position and support a person safely and comfortably. The doctor or hospice nurse may recommend a urinary catheter to protect the skin and to help keep your caregivee/loved one clean and dry. Special equipment may be ordered, such as an alternating pressure mattress for comfort and to protect the skin. The hospice nurse and other care team members may make more frequent visits. The social worker or chaplain may call to see if you would like to meet. If it is within your caregivee/loved one's faith system, a member of the clergy may come to your home to perform "last rites" or other sacred rituals.

Oxygen may be prescribed as a comfort measure. Oxygen does not "cure," but it may provide comfort by creating a sensation of air moving near the nasal passages. An oxygen "mask" is not usually recommended because a mask may be uncomfortable for your caregivee/loved one to wear and may hinder important communication with caregivers and family members. The hospice team may recommend that you place a fan in the room to circulate air and provide comfort in the form of more air moving over and around the caregivee/loved one.

As your caregivee/loved one's disease process continues, they may exhibit a decreased appetite. This is a natural part of the dying process. It may be difficult for some caregivers to have food refused. We have been taught in our society that food provides strength and vitality. Food is also tied to nurturing, socialization, and fellowship. Toward the end of life, the body very naturally requires less food and fewer calories. This may be because it takes a tremendous amount of energy to digest food. Your caregivee/loved one may eat smaller meals served more frequently or a small serving of favorite foods served on a small plate. This may be more appealing to them. They may request a special food and then be unable to eat it. Knowing that this is natural may make this easier to accept. Do not be hurt by your caregivee/loved one's decline in appetite or refusal of food.

A normal, healthy adult is encouraged to "drink a lot of fluids" or have IV fluids, especially when we are ill. This changes at the end of life as well. The body may be calling for fewer fluids because it is an easier and more efficient way for the body to maintain its normal homeostasis or "balance." It's a good idea to have your caregivee/loved one's favorite beverage and water nearby, but you may see that they drink less and less and that they may only sip fluids to keep their mouth moist.

Take comfort in knowing that a sleeping person is usually a comfortable person and if your caregivee/loved one is sleeping more than usual, but waking up alert and oriented, then their symptoms are well managed. As a person moves closer to the end of life, they may sleep more, awaken less often, and be less alert. This may be accompanied by a decreased appetite and a decrease in the amount of fluids that they drink. They may go to the bathroom less often and their urine may become dark in color and perhaps have a strong odor. Your caregivee/loved one should still be having bowel movements, but they may be smaller if they are not eating. They will continue to have bowel movements because the digestive tract continues to work even when the caregivee/loved one has stopped eating.

As Death Approaches

Death is as individual as people's personalities, yet there are commonalities that are seen at the end of life. Breathing changes and non-responsiveness are two of those commonalities. They also might become incontinent and a catheter may be ordered by the doctor for comfort reasons.

You may see some of the following signs and symptoms that will tell you that your caregivee/loved one is nearing their end of life:

Your caregivee/loved one may "withdraw" and sleep for long, or longer, periods of time.

They may awaken and feel refreshed and want to engage in conversation with you. Or, they may awaken and still seem withdrawn and go back into deep sleep again.

Over time, they may communicate less, becoming more weakened. Please realize that it may take too much energy for them to converse. It is strongly believed that the person can still hear you even if non-responsive or in a deep sleep. Remember this and speak kindly and in soft tones. Always assume your caregivee/loved one can hear you and include them in your conversations. Also, try to avoid talking "about" them in their presence. Perhaps recall fun or poignant times that were once shared. Though they may appear unresponsive, they may be able to squeeze your hand.

You may hear or notice irregular breathing. Breathing may be rapid and appear shallow. Or there may be long spaces between breaths. It is not uncommon for a person to breathe in these irregular patterns as death approaches.

You may hear your caregivee/loved one have a gurgling sound in the back of their throat. It may sound as if they need to cough to "clear their throat." This sound is caused when their vocal chords and other throat muscles relax. It has not been found to be uncomfortable to the caregivee/

loved one, but it may be uncomfortable for the family to hear. Knowing what that sound is may ease fear that you may have that the person is uncomfortable.

A person's skin may become cool or cooler to the touch. You may notice that their extremities, such as their hands, feet, arms, and legs, are particularly cool. You may see a purplish or dark coloring to the skin on their extremities as well. This is an indicator that their body systems are beginning to shut down.

Your caregivee/loved one may develop a low fever. This is usually not a concern, but may be treated if they are uncomfortable.

Toward the end of life, you may see your caregivee/loved one breathing through their mouth. This may cause the mouth to become uncomfortable. This is even more true if your caregivee/loved one is on oxygen. Use a lip balm to keep their lips moist and if your caregivee/loved one is on oxygen, ask the hospice nurse about a safe product to moisten lips. Do not use petroleum-based products if a person is on oxygen.

You may also notice that your caregivee/loved one has a diminished ability to close their eyes or to blink.

At the far end of life, the caregivee/loved one's breaths may come at distant intervals. Perhaps 30 seconds or more might pass between breaths. This is a normal indicator of end of life and may indicate that death is near. Hopefully the family and dear friends will have gathered by this time, but if they have not and you desire them to be present, call them. Always notify the hospice team of any significant changes. Sometimes the hospice team can tell you when it is time to gather the person's family and friends. Please do not hesitate to ask your hospice team these types of questions. They are there to guide you.

4. Personal Care Considerations: Care of the dying caregivee/loved one should be extremely gentle. And, as with any person in any setting, always tell them what you are going to do before you do it and what you are doing as you do it. Sometimes, toward the end of life, a person may experience an increase in pain. They may have become very thin and turning them or repositioning them in bed may be very uncomfortable for them. The hospice nurse may recommend that you "pre-medicate" your caregivee/loved one with pain medication a half hour before performing personal care. Ask the hospice nurse about this if you notice that your caregivee/loved one experiences discomfort during daily care. Discomfort may appear as facial grimacing, a furrowed brow, and/or moaning.

Daily mouth care is very important and is a valuable comfort measure. As caregiver, be on the lookout for white spots on the tongue and/or on the sides of the mouth, or a white coating on the tongue. This could indicate that your caregivee/loved one has developed an infection, such as thrush, and you should let the hospice nurse know right away. It can and should be treated. Consider mouth care an important comfort measure.

5. Safety Considerations: Your caregivee/loved one may or may not have a document called a "DNR" (do-not-resuscitate) order. In some states, the DNR document is printed on a very brightly colored paper. This document notifies emergency medical services or technicians (EMS/EMT) that your caregivee/loved one does not want resuscitation measures/chest compressions in the event of an emergency. This document should be prominently displayed in the home near your caregivee/loved one. If you have any questions about a DNR, ask your doctor or any member of the hospice care team.

Your caregivee/loved one may be prescribed strong medications that could be dangerous if not taken exactly as prescribed. Any medication should *always* be kept out of the reach of children and teenagers.

6. When to Call the Doctor, Nurse, or Care Team:

- Caregivee/loved one is showing any signs of discomfort.
- Caregivee/loved one has a fever.
- Caregivee/loved one is showing any sign of uncontrolled pain such as grimacing, a furrowed brow, and/or moaning during movement or while being still.
- Caregivee/loved one has increased confusion.
- Caregivee/loved one is anxious.
- Caregivee/loved one is unable to sleep (fall asleep or stay asleep).
- Caregivee/loved one is expressing spiritual distress.
- Caregivee/loved one is showing any signs of depression.
- Caregivee/loved one is experiencing hallucinations.
- Caregivee/loved one's family or friends are experiencing or demonstrating behavior that may be disruptive to the caregivee/loved one.
- Caregivee/loved one has fallen.
- If you have concerns, or see change that disturbs you, call the hospice nurse.

These are examples only. Your caregivee/loved one might relay to you changes or concerns that vary from those listed here and those concerns should be addressed with your care team.

7. Comfort Considerations: The goal of hospice and palliative care is comfort.

The hospice team works with you to address your caregivee/loved one's physical, mental, and spiritual comfort. As a caregiver, providing comfort sometimes means "the small things." Small things are sometimes easily overlooked. Having regular bowel movements may seem like a small thing, but it is actually a very important aspect of caregivee/loved one comfort.

If your caregivee/loved one is on any pain medication, they can and, in many cases, do cause constipation. Sometimes they may need to take a stool softener or laxative for as long as they are on pain medications. It is always better to prevent a problem than to correct a problem, and this is never more true than when it comes to pain medicines and constipation. We encourage you not to be shy about asking your caregivee/loved one about their bowel habits and call the hospice nurse if their bowels have not moved for three days. Please remember that this is true even if they are not eating very much. When a hospice caregivee/loved one becomes constipated it can lead to extreme discomfort. If the hospice nurse has not spoken to you about laxatives, please ask.

If your caregivee/loved one seems to be unable to catch their breath, as may happen with persons who are dying from a respiratory illness (COPD, lung cancer), contact the hospice nurse and ask for suggestions to control the symptom that you are seeing. It is likely that you will already have been taught how to best address this symptom, known as "air hunger," but if you not been taught, if the change is sudden, or if you have any concerns, call!

The hospice team may provide you with small sponges on a stick that can be moistened and used gently in your caregivee's mouth to keep the mouth moist and comfortable. Again, it is often the small things that provide comfort and a dry mouth needs to be addressed early, often, and consistently. Toward the end of life, you may see your caregivee/loved one breathing through their mouth and this can cause the mouth to become very dry and uncomfortable. This is even more true if your caregivee/loved one is on oxygen. Do not use petroleum-based products if a person is on oxygen. Provide drinks to sip, consider using a drinking straw, and ask your hospice team if ice chips or hard candy to suck on would be a suitable comfort measure for your caregivee/loved one. Use a lip balm to keep their lips moist. If your caregivee/loved one is on oxygen, ask the hospice nurse to recommend a safe product to moisten lips.

Use pillows of varying sizes, as needed, as a comfort measure. Pillows or rolled up face cloths, a folded towel, or blankets might be used to prop up their head, arms, or legs, or be placed behind the knees. The hospice nurse and/or hospice aide can show you how to do this to support the person's weight and, in some cases, reduce swelling and protect your caregivee/loved one's skin.

As people approach the end of life, they may have a diminished ability to close their eyes or blink. This can cause dry eyes and can be very uncomfortable. The hospice nurse may suggest using normal saline eye drops to be gently placed in the person's eyes as often as needed. Small comfort measures such as this mean a great deal. Ask the hospice nurse to demonstrate how to administer eye drops if you are having difficulty. For further recommendations related to caregivee/loved one comfort, ask the hospice nurse and hospice aide. They may know other small, but important, ways to keep your caregivee/loved one comfortable.

8. Special Considerations: For many families, end of life is a time for family, friends, and loved ones to gather but it also may not be depending on your caregivee/loved one's wishes. During the time that the hospice team has been working with you, there may have been conversations initiated in which the caregivee/loved one was able to express their thoughts and wishes as they pertain to family relationships. These are considered sacred times and sacred conversations. These conversations will help you gauge if your caregivee/loved one would like all of their family at the bedside or only a few close people, such as friends. As much as possible, allow and honor these wishes. The room of a dying person is usually a place where great respect is demonstrated. The noise level should be kept low. Televisions should be turned off. If your caregivee/loved one had a love of a special kind of music, perhaps have that playing softly in the background. Again, and as always, base all of this on their wishes.

Most or many people do not want to die alone. This can be considered generally true. Sometimes, though, the person waits for someone to leave the room. They may not want to hurt a loved one's feelings or cause stress to a person they love. When that special person comes back into the room, they see the caregivee/loved one resting and at peace. Some caregivers have spent hours or perhaps even days at the bedside of their dying loved one only to leave the room for a few minutes and, while they were out of the room, their loved one died. Many believe that people at the end-of-life choose the time they die.

Another consideration is that some people will wait to see a loved one before they die. They may be extremely withdrawn and sleeping much of the time. When the person they have been waiting for arrives, you may see your caregivee/loved one have a period of clarity and alertness, withdraw again, and then die.

Some people may set a "goal" for themselves, such as wanting to attend a daughter's wedding or a grandchild's graduation. They may attend the event and have a grand day and appear full of energy. After attending the event, the person may then start to withdraw and begin a more active dying process.

Sometimes a caregivee/loved one may need to be given verbal permission to "go." They may be especially concerned about a particular family member, a spouse, a child in need, or have a business concern. They may need to hear words such as "It is ok to go. We will take good care of _____ and see to it that (they/it) is/are well cared for."

The following "Five Tasks for End-of-Life" seek to reconcile relationships between friends or families and their loved ones at the end of life. The following tasks may be spoken to the caregivee/loved one by persons close to them, and vice-versa; the caregivee/loved one may speak them to their loved ones. This can be a meaningful exercise for the person, for the caregiver, and/or family members and it may help ease or lessen the grieving process after death. It is not "mandatory," it does not have to be done perfectly or even at all. But if this kind of task appeals to you or if you think that it would be meaningful for your caregivee/loved one, ask them these words or accomplish these tasks in whatever way makes sense to you (or to whoever is doing them). Perhaps it is done silently, in a prayerful way, or spoken to your caregivee/loved one during a time of quiet communication or during personal care. Perhaps each family member spends time alone with the caregivee/loved one and speaks or discusses these tasks. The tasks are as follows:

1. Asking for forgiveness (please forgive me).
2. Offering forgiveness (I forgive you).
3. Offering thanks (thank you).
4. Offering love (I love you).
5. Saying goodbye.

(Morrow, 2014; also see the *The Four Things That Matter Most: A Book About Living* by Ira Byock)

These tasks bring us to the discussion of difficult and/or sensitive family matters. When a person is dying and family gathers, it is a remarkable and sacred time. These gatherings can bring family healing and expressions of true goodness. Sometimes, sadly, old family wounds can be opened, though. If this is the case, drama can occur. Try to limit this type of drama in the presence of your dying loved one. Bring peace and gentility to the bedside of one who is dying. If you have thoughts or concerns about this, such as a particularly disruptive or otherwise troubled family member, contact the hospice nurse or social worker.

9. Special Instructions Given to You by the Doctor, Nurse, or Care Team:

_____

_____

_____

_____

_____

_____

_____

_____

_____

10. Resources:

- A good book about living life to the fullest, especially in our personal relationships, is *The Four Things That Matter Most: A Book About Living* by Ira Byock.
- A good book about cutting funeral costs, and what goes on inside funeral homes, is *Profits of Death: An Insider Exposes the Death Care Industries* by Darryl J. Roberts.
- Support for People with Oral and Head and Neck Cancer is a support group for caregivee/loved ones and families suffering from this cancer that also has local chapters throughout the United States: https://www.spohnc.org
- The Order of the Good Death seeks to make death a part of life, they encourage us to accept that death is a natural part of life to help ease the anxiety surrounding death: http://www.orderofthegooddeath.com/
- A classic book about end of life, Elisabeth Kubler-Ross' *On Death and Dying: What the Dying Have to Teach Doctors, Nurses, Clergy and Their Own Families* explains the five

stages of death and grief you may have heard of before: denial, anger, bargaining, depression, and acceptance.

- The Diane Rehm Show has featured many stories about hospice and end-of-life care including "The Rise of the For-Profit Hospice Industry" (http://thedianerehmshow.org/shows/2015-01-15/the_rise_of_the_for_profit_hospice_industry), "Hospice and End-of-Life Care" (http://thedianerehmshow.org/shows/2000-06-22/hospice-and-end-life-care), "Facing Death: Choosing Quality of Life Over Aggressive Treatment" (http://thedianerehmshow.org/shows/2012-04-16/facing-death-choosing-quality-life-over-aggressive-treatment).

- The *Washington Post* offers a "Consumer guide to hospice," which compares hospices in your area based on things like size, accreditation, how long they have been in business, and who owns them: http://www.washingtonpost.com/wp-srv/special/business/hospice-quality/

- The Health Affairs Blog featured a story from Amy Berman about her perspective on treatment for cancer: http://healthaffairs.org/blog/2014/05/22/narrative-matters-the-next-chapter-amy-berman-reflects-on-living-life-in-my-own-way/

- There is also a talk from Amy Berman on the NIH's website: http://videocast.nih.gov/summary.asp?Live=11519&bhcp=1

- The National Cancer Institute offers many end-of-life resources, including "Preparing for the End of Life" (http://www.cancer.gov/cancertopics/coping/end-of-life), "Palliative Care in Cancer" (http://www.cancer.gov/cancertopics/advanced-cancer/care-choices/palliative-care-fact-sheet).

- Aging with Dignity is an organization that offers many resources for those facing the end of life, including the "Five Wishes," a popular living will option that is legally recognized in 42 states and available in 27 languages: https://www.agingwithdignity.org/five-wishes.php
- *Caring for the Human Spirit* magazine is from the Health Care Chaplaincy Network and aims to promote the integration of spiritual care in healthcare: https://www.healthcarechaplaincy.org/caring-for-the-human-spirit-magazine.html
- The Health Care Chaplaincy also offers numerous resources, including veteran-focused chaplaincy (http://chaplaincareforveterans.org/), cancer-centered chaplaincy (http://cantbelieveihavecancer.org/), and "Chat with a Chaplain" by either email, phone, or video (http://chaplainsonhand.org/cms/get-help.html).

References

American Cancer Society. (2014). Where is hospice care given? http://www.cancer.org/treatment/findingandpayingfortreatment/choosingyourtreatmentteam/hospicecare/hospice-care-settings

Centers for Disease Control and Prevention (CDC). (2013). Trends in Inpatient Hospital Deaths: National Hospital Discharge Survey, 2000–2010. Retrieved from http://www.cdc.gov/nchs/data/databriefs/db118.htm

MedlinePlus. (n.d.). What is palliative care? Retrieved from http://www.nlm.nih.gov/medlineplus/ency/patientinstructions/000536.htm

Morrow, A. (2014). The Five Tasks of Dying: Finding Closure and Peace at the End of Life. Retrieved from http://dying.about.com/od/thedyingprocess/a/5_tasks_dying.htm

National Hospice and Palliative Care Organization (NHPCO). (2014). NHPCO's Facts and Figures: Hospice Care in America, 2014 Edition. Retrieved from http://www.nhpco.org/sites/default/files/public/Statistics_Research/2014_Facts_Figures.pdf

PBS. (2010). Facing Death: Facts & Figures. Retrieved from http://www
.pbs.org/wgbh/pages/frontline/facing-death/facts-and-figures/

Temel, J., Greer, J. A., Muzikansky, A., Gallagher, R. N., Admane, S.,
Jackson, V. A., . . . Lynch, T. J. (2010). Early Palliative Care for Patients
with Metastatic Non–Small-Cell Lung Cancer. *The New England Journal of Medicine*, 363:733–742.

OLDER ADULT CARE

1. Introduction: Most caregiving is directed toward older adults. For purposes of this section, an older adult will be defined as a person over 70 years old. You may have heard the saying "70" is the new "50." What this means is that aging, more and more, is just a number. Of course, we all live a finite amount of time on this earth, but baby boomers and the "oldest old" are changing ideas and beliefs about aging. There was a time when 60 and 65 were considered "old." This is no longer the case! Especially for active and healthy older adults. And the numbers tell the story. "In 2010, 40 million people age 65 and over lived in the United States, accounting for 13 percent of the total population. The older population grew from 3 million in 1900 to 40 million in 2010. The oldest-old population (those age 85 and over) grew from just over 100,000 in 1900 to 5.5 million in 2010. The "Baby Boomers" (those born between 1946 and 1964) started turning 65 in 2011" (AgingStats.gov, n.d.). The number of older people will increase dramatically over the coming years: "the number of older people will increase dramatically during the 2010–2030 period. The older population in 2030 is projected to be twice as large as their counterparts in 2000, growing from 35 million to 72 million and representing nearly 20 percent of the total U.S. population" (AgingStats.gov, n.d.). Just walk down the street, visit Florida or Arizona, or take a cruise—it is easy to see that the aging are all around and, if we are not there already, we will soon be joining them! Because there are sometimes three generations of older adults living with and caring for the oldest old, this has huge implications for care and caregivers. There are many physiological changes that are associated with aging that are a normal part of the aging process. This chapter focuses on the oldest old, as they have the most care needs, and seeks to highlight some of the areas that are of particular importance when caring for this very special caregivee/loved one population.

2. General Information: Many older adults have a complexity of health problems that impact their daily lives and functions. They may be "chronically ill," meaning having a long-lasting or recurrent illness or health problem. They may also need help with numerous tasks that were taken for granted when they were well. For example, an older adult may have been discharged from the hospital back to home. Home is defined as wherever the person lives. This could be a son and daughter-in-law's home, an independent care apartment, or their longtime house where they wed and raised a family over the years. In any case, once back home, the older adult may have trouble with what are called "activities of daily living." These are just what they sound like—the things/activities/tasks that must be done daily for grooming, hygiene, and overall self-care. These include such daily activities as bathing, showering, dressing, the ability to transfer or move from a bed to a chair, eating and drinking, and meal preparation and serving. It also includes other bodily functions, such as being able to urinate and get to the bathroom when needed.

How the person does or performs these activities is also important for safety reasons; particularly if the person lives alone. Sometimes the person may be able to physically do these things, but needs to be "cued" (reminded exactly what to do like telling them to take a bite, chew, swallow, etc.). Perhaps because of Alzheimer's disease or another dementia, they may be unable to remember to do such seemingly simple, everyday tasks.

There are many other tasks that one must also do in order to remain safe at home and live independently. These are called "Instrumental Activities of Daily Living" and include such things as: being able to take medications correctly; maintaining the home (housework or caring for a pet or pets); being able to manage money; preparing, cooking, and cleaning up after meals; being able to use the telephone; and other activities. Just consider what one must do every day to care for themselves and their homes—it is a lot! Now, imagine that you are a 96 year old man and live alone. This is where the problems and safety risks are.

Things to consider include realizing that the senses generally deteriorate or diminish with age. This means that hearing may become less acute, so they might be very hard of hearing or deaf. Their sense of smell may diminish and so they may be less able to smell smoke. This ability to smell also has implications for nutrition as the taste of food may also decrease so they may decrease the amount of calories they consume. Some older adults may say that foods and spices "do not taste the same." This sometimes is noted when an older adult tries to put lots of salt on their food or they only want sweet-tasting things like chocolate or cherry jelly.

In addition, the older persons mobility and functional balance may also decrease and so they may be more prone to falls or other mishaps. They may also have severe vision loss and need glasses. Other changes to be aware of include ones that cannot "be seen." One of the most dangerous is that their bones can lose "density," which can cause osteoporosis. Osteoporosis literally means "porous bone" (PubMed Health, n.d.). "This disease is characterized by too little bone formation, excessive bone loss, or a combination of both, leading to bone fragility and an increased risk of fractures of the hip, spine and wrist" (PubMed Health, n.d.). This is more of a problem because people "over the age of 70 are more likely to have low bone density. Plus, the risk of falling increases in old age, which then also makes fractures more likely" (PubMed Health, n.d.). This bone condition can also contribute to brittle bones that can fracture, or break easily, with a fall or simple pressure.

Another area of change in the older person is the skin, which can become tissue-paper thin. This literally thin skin can tear or break down or bruise very easily. The oldest old also may feel cold and have a need to have the heat to be on or set higher than the younger people living in the same home. This is seen when other people are complaining of the heat (either outside or in the house) and the older adult has a sweater on or a shawl or blanket on their lap or over their knees. Some accommodation must be made when these frail elders are cold. Try to keep them as comfortable as possible and try to keep them from catching a cold—or being cold.

Frailty or being frail is also a big problem. Frailty is a cluster or compilation of factors or conditions that carry additional risks of morbidity and mortality. Though hard to define, "frailty" looks and sounds like just what it is. Let's look again at that 96-year-old gentleman that was mentioned above. He is very thin (though he still eats well), stands stooped over his cane, has noticeably tissue-paper-thin skin on his arms with some bruising noted, walks very slowly, and looks at the ground while walking. In addition, it takes an inordinately long (and slow) time for him to be able to stand up from a sitting position—even from a chair that is high for this purpose and has sturdy arms—to help him get up safely. Any change in the environment or change in the structure of the day or the setting can be a risky endeavor. The adult children help guide him with a hand under his arm and gently lead him to where he is going. With frailty there are a cluster of known or identified risk factors. These might include falls, infections, or functional incontinence (they cannot get to the bathroom quickly and so may be incontinent). They may also not want to drink fluids, even when offered, because they do not want to have to get up and walk into the bathroom— again, all movement is an effort and takes what little reserve these frail elders have.

If this sounds like your parents or grandparents—they may be frail. They may have some confusion and are generally thought to be at risk for falls, hospitalization, and death. Watch them with love and tenderness, but like a hawk! They might also need total care assistance for personal care activities. For example, an adult child or an aide must care for the person and cue them to shower, brush their teeth, or otherwise maintain good hygiene. This amount of frailty also assumes that an aide or the family shops; prepares meals; sets up for breakfast, lunch, and dinner and serves food; and many other daily routines for care and safety. What might be a minor change in the environment to you and me could be a major stressor or problem for these frail oldest old. Every day they live on the edge of a fall or other untoward event. For all these safety reasons, a nutritious diet; socialization; ongoing exercise to maintain the older adult's strength, balance, and gait; and a safe home environment are all key components of supporting, nurturing care. Maintaining the older adult's independence for as long as possible is the goal.

Of course, the oldest old are the cohort of elders that are moving toward the end of their lives—so make their time on earth as fun and pleasurable as it can be. Try to make every day the best it can be—if there are foods they like, make them; if they like to play cards, play cards; if there is a veterans group meeting in your community and they are also a veteran from that era, bring him or her. It is good to know that sometimes those longer term memories are more accessible to these elders than what they did yesterday or last week. It all depends—but try and have some fun in their lives every day. Make these special memories while you can! Regardless of these or other health problems, some older adults may be set in their beliefs and values. It is very important to respect and honor their decisions to do things in their own way unless they are not appropriate or safe.

Readers are also referred to Chapter Six: Safety in the Home: The Most Frequent Health Care Setting of Choice! as well as the individual Special Patient Populations that are most appropriate for your caregivee/loved one. This might include chapters such as "Alzheimer's Disease and Dementia Care," "Arthritis Care," "Bedbound Care (Care of the Immobilized or Bedridden Patient)," "Diabetes Care," "End-of-Life Care," "Urinary and Incontinence Care," or others.

3. General Goals for Care: Bottom line goals: Keep your caregivee/loved one clean, safe, and comfortable with nutrition and hydration as they choose. Make sure that safe assistance of activities of daily living are provided and the caregivee/loved one is safely and lovingly cared for. Other goals are those related to the unique interests of the older adult and the fun activities of their choosing. This may be old movies, time with grandchildren, spending time with photos or scrapbooks as a part of life review, and many others—as individualized as the interests and life of your caregivee/loved one!

4. Personal Care Considerations: As always, tell the person what you are going to do before you do it and what you are doing as you do it. For example, if your caregivee/loved one is incontinent, try not to embarrass them and respect their need for privacy as much as possible. If appropriate, perhaps remind them to use the bathroom just before their usual time if you have noticed a pattern, for example, every two hours during the day. Providing reminders for the caregivee/loved one, using adult language, and keeping the pathway to the bathroom well lit and free of clutter may also help reduce incontinence. Also remind them to use the bathroom before you are taking the caregivee/loved one out—such as to a restaurant or a senior center for some activity. You might also consider using adult briefs for privacy and comfort. Sometimes a frail elder person will prefer these, especially at nighttime.

Skin care is another important area for older adults, particularly if they are bedridden or sit in one position for lengthy periods of time. Nutritional deficiencies, immobility, and illness can contribute to the risk of skin breaking down and forming pressure ulcers or sores. Changes in the skin should be reported to the doctor or the nurse. In addition, many of the oldest old have arthritis, and sometimes in the mornings it may be more painful to move their joints during bathing, for example. Let the caregivee/loved one tell you how to move them and when they are "ready" to move. During the bath or shower, inspect your caregivee/loved one's skin for any breakdown, bruising, skin tears, redness, or other changes. Be very gentle when moving or turning those who have tissue-paper-thin skin if it is very fragile and tears easily. If there is a skin tear, place a bandage over the area and ask the home care nurse what else you can do to prevent further injury. Use a "pull sheet" to gently reposition your caregivee/loved one if in bed. Again, notify the nurse or the doctor for any new skin problems. For more information, see "Bedbound Care (Care of the Immobilized or Bedridden Patient)."

Communications during bathing and other personal care activities are important, especially for safety, such as when your caregivee/loved one may be asked to sit on the shower chair or stand up and hold on to the grab bars for safety. This can be more problematic with a confused or hearing-impaired caregivee/loved one. And—to make things more dangerous—their glasses and hearing aids may be off while bathing and so they cannot see or hear as well. So always be careful in the bathroom. Because personal care takes time and is very personal and intimate, this can be a time for meaningful communication and time together. And this is the time that some people like to reminisce about the past and share memories. Listen attentively and respect your caregivee/loved one by not talking "baby talk" or raising your voice. It is more helpful to rephrase what you are saying when a person is hard of hearing or speak more slowly and clearly rather than speaking louder. Assist with cleaning of glasses, hearing aids, and other items, such as assistive devices like canes and walkers, too.

5. Safety Considerations: Some older adults may have poor balance, poor core muscle strength, and/or slow reflexes and are more at risk for fractures and other injuries from falls. In addition, multiple medications may increase the chance for falls. Caregivers are referred to Chapter Six: Safety in the Home: The Most Frequent Health Care Setting of Choice! where there is a discussion about medications, safety and older adults. Falls could possibly be avoided by clearing the household walkways of clutter when possible. Be sure to keep assistive/adaptive devices close to your caregivee/loved one, such as a walker, quad cane, or other safety equipment. Keep the phone within the person's reach for safety. Cell phones have made this a little easier because of the mobility of the phone—then you just need to remind your caregivee/loved one to keep it in their pocket! Some older adults who live alone, or may be alone during the day, might consider a personal emergency response system (PERS) in case they would need help. If your caregivee/loved one has this, encourage them to wear their button or bracelet as required for this technology to work. Also, if you go out, remind your caregivee/loved one that they should not answer the door, not climb on anything to reach for something, and to use their assistive devices at all times. If they are forgetful, consider a notecard with big print that reads "Did you take your medications?" One suggestion is to place their medications for the day in the same special container in the same place for their use each morning and have another note that says what the month, day/date, and year is. These kinds of reminders and visual cues are very helpful for older adults with memory problems.

6. When to Call the Doctor, the Nurse, or Care Team:
These are only possible examples and NOT an inclusive list. Please remember that calling *before* a situation becomes a bigger problem is always best. It's better to catch problems when they are relatively small. It is much harder to address "big" problems.

- Caregivee/loved one has fallen.
- Caregivee/loved one has new or increased confusion or other behavioral changes (this can be a sign of an infection, for one example).
- Caregivee/loved one exhibits signs or symptoms of a cold or the flu (influenza), the flu can be very dangerous and deadly to the oldest old.
- Caregivee/loved one has changes in skin, appetite, alertness, orientation.
- Caregivee/loved one is coughing, has a fever, or other symptoms that are not usual.
- Caregivee/loved one no longer recognizes loved ones or they exhibit wandering behavior.
- Caregivee/loved one cannot be awakened.
- Any other change, complication, or concern that you or the caregivee/loved one may have. When in doubt, call!

These are examples only. Your caregivee/loved one might relay to you changes or concerns that vary from those listed here and those concerns should be addressed with your care team.

7. Comfort Considerations: Comfort for your caregivee/ loved one can mean physical, mental, spiritual, or any combination of those kinds of comfort. As a caregiver, providing comfort sometimes means "the small things." Small things are sometimes easily overlooked. Having regular bowel movements may seem like a small thing, but it is actually a very large part of comfort. If your caregivee/loved one is on any pain medication, they can and, in many cases, do cause constipation. You may need to keep track of their bowel movements to prevent constipation. If this is the case, call the doctor who may suggest a stool softener or other medication.

8. Special Considerations: Older adults, and especially the oldest old, can get dehydrated very easily. This can occur from not drinking enough fluids, taking certain medications (one example is a diuretic, also called a "water pill"), extreme heat, and other reasons. Dehydration and/or an infection can cause falls or confusion in some people. A word about medication: because the body systems slow down in older adults, and especially in the oldest old, there is a saying about medications with this caregivee/loved one population to "start low and go slow" since frailty already makes some older people very at-risk for falls or other problems. Protect your caregivee/ loved one and be very observant after new medications are started. Overall, the best care for the oldest old is keeping them comfortable, warm and safe, while being kind and honoring their wishes. They should also not be alone for extended periods of time. All people, regardless of age and health, need socialization, mental stimulation, and company.

9. Special Instructions Given to You by the Doctor, Nurse, or Care Team:

_____

_____

_____

_____

_____

_____

_____

_____

_____

10. Resources:

- NIHSeniorHealth offers many resources for older adults, including ones on the benefits of staying active and exercising, if possible: http://nihseniorhealth.gov/exerciseforolder adults/healthbenefits/01.html
- MedlinePlus has an information page on osteoporosis: http://www.nlm.nih.gov/medlineplus/osteoporosis.html
- The Centers for Disease Control and Prevention (CDC) offers a page on healthy aging with resources including emergency preparedness, chronic disease management, and the healthy brain initiative: http://www.cdc.gov/aging/
- HealthyPeople.gov has a page dedicated to older adult health with resources on chronic diseases common in older adults and statistics on older Americans: https://www .healthypeople.gov/2020/topics-objectives/topic/older-adults
- The World Health Organization (WHO) offers a fact sheet on mental health and older adults: http://www.who.int/ mediacentre/factsheets/fs381/en/

- The PACE (Program of All-inclusive Care for the Elderly), from Medicare and Medicaid, aims to help people meet their needs in the community so they do not have to enter a long-term care facility if possible: http://www.medicare.gov/your-medicare-costs/help-paying-costs/pace/pace.html
- The Eldercare Locator from the Department of Health and Human Services offers a search tool for finding help for your caregivee/loved one based on the problem they may be facing, like long term care needs or nutrition, and your location: eldercare.gov or 1-800-677-1116
- Adult Protective Services has offices across the country to help you if you think your caregivee/loved one is being taken advantage of or abused. To locate a location near you: http://www.napsa-now.org/get-help/help-in-your-area
- The American Psychological Association (APA) has information about "Older Adults' Health and Age-Related Changes" on their site: http://www.apa.org/pi/aging/resources/guides/older.aspx
- The National Institute of Mental Health (NIH) also has information about "Older Adults and Mental Health": http://www.nimh.nih.gov/health/topics/older-adults-and-mental-health/index.shtml

References

AgingStats.gov. (n.d.). Population. Retrieved from http://www.agingstats.gov/main_site/data/2012_documents/population.aspx

PubMed Health. (n.d.). Osteoporosis. Retrieved from http://www.ncbi.nlm.nih.gov/pubmedhealth/PMHT0024680/

STROKE CARE (CEREBROVASCULAR ACCIDENT)

1. Introduction: Strokes occur when the blood supply to the brain is interrupted, causing brain cell tissue to die. A stroke is a medical emergency! There are two kinds of strokes. An ischemic (is-skeem-ik) stroke happens when a blood vessel becomes blocked or clogged and oxygen-rich blood stops nourishing that area of the brain. A hemorrhagic (hem-or-ah-jik) stroke occurs when a blood vessel breaks and there is bleeding within the brain. Whether ischemic or hemorrhagic, brain damage begins to occur in the immediate area within minutes. Sometimes the blood flow to the brain is only briefly interrupted, and when this happens, the event is called a "TIA," which stands for Transient Ischemic Attack. TIAs are commonly referred to as "mini strokes." TIAs still need to be investigated immediately and should not be ignored. Persons who have had a previous stroke and/or cardiac disease are more at risk for stroke. The risk for another stroke is greatest shortly after a stroke and this risk decreases over time.

Strokes are most common in people over the age of 65 (National Institute of Neurological Disorders and Stroke [NINDS], 2013). Women tend to have strokes more often than men, and have a higher incidence of death from strokes (The American Stroke Association, 2012). Risk factors for stroke include obesity, diabetes, high blood pressure, chronic kidney disease, heart disease, smoking, TIAs, and artery disease, such as atherosclerosis—especially atherosclerosis in the carotid arteries, which supply blood to the brain. Atherosclerosis is described later in this chapter. Blood disorders, such as sickle cell anemia or other diseases that cause blood to thicken, might also increase the risk of blood clots and therefore stroke. Having a family history of strokes and some congenital (from birth) abnormalities may increase the risk of stroke as well.

A person who has had a stroke may have tests to determine the type and severity of the stroke. Immediately following a stroke they may be treated with medications and/or surgery. Depending on the severity of the symptoms and the deficits incurred, the caregivee/loved one may go to a post-stroke rehabilitation unit after they are initially diagnosed and treated. Post-stroke treatment often includes rehabilitation therapy, stroke prevention education, medication, and lifestyle changes.

According to the Centers for Disease Control and Prevention (CDC), in 2012, 6.4 million adults who experienced a stroke did not require institutionalization (CDC, 2013). Between 2009 and 2010, 3.7 million caregivee/loved ones were seen in physician's offices, outpatient departments and emergency departments with stroke as their primary diagnosis (CDC, 2013). In 2013 there were 128,978 deaths from stroke, ranking stroke as the number 5 cause of death in the United States (CDC, 2013).

You may also refer to other chapters in this book such as: "Bedbound Care (Care of the Immobilized or Bedridden Patient)," "Cardiac Care," Diabetes Care," "End-of-Life Care," and "Older Adult Care."

2. General Information: Depending upon what part of the brain was affected, a stroke may cause paralysis or muscle weakness on one side of the body. Paralysis on one side of the body is called hemiplegia and one-sided weakness is called hemiparesis. After a stroke in which one side of the body is affected, the person may demonstrate a loss of awareness of the weakened side. They may ignore or even forget their weaker side, and this phenomenon can put them at risk for hurting themselves. In addition, the decreased sense of feeling pain from a stroke may make them more susceptible to injury or pressure ulcers. They may also have a lesser visual field on the side that has been affected.

Thinking or cognitive skills may be affected and the person may have a lessened ability to think clearly or to concentrate. Your caregivee/loved one may demonstrate emotional mood swings as a result of a stroke. They may cry more easily or laugh inappropriately and post-stroke persons often experience depression. They may also have problems communicating. They may have difficulty understanding what they are hearing and they may have difficulty speaking or even lose the ability to speak. When a person loses the ability to speak, this is called aphasia. Aphasia can also affect the ability to listen, read, and write. Dysphasia is an impairment in the ability to speak or communicate.

A stroke can affect the person's ability to swallow; one or both sides of the mouth may have become weakened and/or lose feeling. If this is the case, the caregivee/loved one may have difficulty swallowing safely, and could be at risk for choking. Pain can result from a stroke as well. People who have had a stroke may experience uncomfortable numbness and tingling sensations of their affected limb(s) and some persons experience intense chronic (long-term) pain if the stroke damaged specific areas of their nervous system.

Imagine everything that your brain does and you will

quickly see that the effects of stroke can be extremely varied and far reaching.

In the course of recovering from a stroke, your caregivee/ loved one may be seen by many different health care professionals. Guided by the physician, often a neurologist, members of this "interdisciplinary team" may include: registered nurses, physical therapists, occupational therapists, speech/ language pathologists, social workers, psychologists, and recreational therapists.

A registered nurse (RN) may specialize in post-stroke care, medication management, and education of the disease process. A physical therapist plays an invaluable role in the stroke survivor's rehabilitation, addressing problems of balance, coordination, and movement. An occupational therapist can help the person adapt at home so that they may regain as much independence as possible. A speech-language pathologist addresses speech, language, and/or swallowing difficulties. A social worker often helps by providing information and facilitating decisions about various facilities, transportation arrangements, financial issues, and support networks. A psychologist may help diagnosis and address mental and emotional issues. A recreational therapist might help the person "re-create" activities that they enjoyed prior to the stroke, perhaps card playing or bird watching. Other professionals may be involved as well, such as a urologist if the person has bladder or urinary issues or a dietitian or nutritionist to make suggestions for person-specific, safe nutritional meals. If the caregivee/loved one needs leg or other braces for support, they may meet with an orthotist. If the caregivee/love one will be going back to work or school, they may see a vocational counselor. And, of course, your caregivee/loved one and yourself are the keystone members of the interdisciplinary care team! The caregiver is the person who knows the caregivee/loved one best, and knows their pre-stroke functional abilities and personality.

After a person has a stroke, doctors might use imaging tests such as a CAT Scan (computerized axial tomography) and/or an MRI (magnetic resonance imaging)—special types of medical imaging—to look at the brain. A stroke may be visible on these tests, but TIAs usually are not. An "angiogram" may be performed to indicate which vessel is blocked or bleeding. The doctor performs an angiogram test by inserting a catheter (tube) and dye into a blood vessel in the body, usually in the arm or groin. Often, medication is given to relax the person before this procedure, but they remains awake. Doctors may test electrical brain activity and function by performing an "electroencephalogram," a test that uses small flat metal discs attached to the scalp. They might also test the brain's blood flow to detect blockages using blood flow tests that are not invasive, but use sonography, or sonograms. If the doctors think that a blood clot came from the heart, they may perform an echocardiogram, a non-invasive sonogram test that can provide two and three dimensional images of the heart. They may also perform a sonogram of the carotid arteries, to detect blockages. Their goal is to find where blockages occurred, and where they may occur again, in order to decrease the risk of another, or "recurrent," stroke. Be aware that your caregivee/loved one may be prescribed low-dose aspirin and antiplatelet drugs to decrease the risk of a recurrent stroke.

Controlling risk factors might decrease the risk of a stroke. It is especially important to control the symptoms of high blood pressure, heart disease, and diabetes. High blood pressure, also called hypertension, is often caused by atherosclerosis and is the primary cause of stroke. Atherosclerosis is a build-up of waxy-like, fatty deposits called plaque. Plaque can build up inside the blood vessels that supply blood to all parts of the body, including the brain. It can cause stiffening and narrowing of the blood vessels. This "hardening of the arteries" can happen anywhere in the body. If severe, it causes restricted blood flow and blood clots. There is a strong correlation between diets high in saturated fats and low in fiber and atherosclerosis (Kratz, 2005; Harvard School of Public Health Nutrition Source, n.d.).

High blood pressure usually has no symptoms, but it can cause serious problems such as heart disease, kidney problems, and stroke. Heart diseases such as heart attack, heart failure, and atrial fibrillation can also lead to stroke. And people who have diabetes are often at a greater risk for stroke because they can have other stroke risk factors, such as atherosclerosis (hardened or clogged blood vessels). Medical treatment, a healthy diet, and exercise are essential to diabetes management. If your caregivee/loved one has diabetes, the diabetes educator or endocrinologist (a doctor who deals with conditions related to glands and hormones, like diabetes and thyroid diseases) should also be considered as members of the post-stroke management team.

Taking care of one body system or illness helps to take care of the others. Here is an example: Poor eating habits and smoking are two lifestyle choices that can lead to atherosclerosis. Atherosclerosis can lead to heart disease and heart disease can cause blood to pool and clot in the heart. These clots can be "thrown off" into the circulatory system, which has narrowed veins and arteries because of atherosclerosis. The clot can travel to the brain, become trapped in a narrowed blood vessel, cause a blockage, and cause a stroke. As you can see, the different body systems and illnesses interplay, interact, and affect each other. Adopting healthy lifestyle habits such as eating a healthy diet, losing weight (if recommended), quitting smoking, exercising regularly, and taking medications as prescribed can help all systems of the body and may lessen the risk of stroke.

In an effort to prevent stroke, doctors sometimes recommend a procedure called a carotid endarterectomy (CEA). During this procedure, the physician removes plaque from the carotid arteries, which are located on either side of the neck. To learn more about carotid endarterectomy, visit http://www.nhlbi.nih.gov/health/health-topics/topics/carend. A CEA may be recommended to reduce the risk of stroke or for persons who have a history of TIAs. TIAs can have all of the symptoms of a stroke, but they typically last less than five minutes and are a warning of a stroke. TIAs are not strokes, but they mimic many of the same symptoms, although the symptoms often last less than two hours. TIAs may indicate that a stroke is coming. Sometimes during a CEA the doctor may place a "stent" or tube in the artery to keep the artery open and prevent further clots from forming. For more information on TIAs visit: http://www.nlm.nih.gov/medlineplus/ency/article/000730.htm

Another procedure that a physician may recommend to someone with carotid artery disease is called carotid angioplasty. In this procedure, the doctor uses a catheter to insert a balloon into the artery and, once in place, inflates it to push the plaque back against the artery wall. A stent may be placed

during this procedure as well. For more information on carotid angioplasty visit: http://www.nlm.nih.gov/medlineplus/
ency/article/002953.htm.

Medicines that your caregivee/loved one may take after a
stroke might include blood thinners or "anticoagulants" as
well as other medications to treat any underlying diseases that
may have contributed to the stroke. Blood thinning medication is taken to lessen the chance of a blood clot forming.
Other medications to control high blood pressure and treat
heart disease may be prescribed if necessary. Post-stroke rehabilitation might be part of your caregivee/loved one's treatment plan too, depending upon their symptoms.

The goal of "post-stroke rehab" is to help your caregivee/
loved one become as independent as possible. Physical, occupational, and speech therapists work with caregivee/loved
ones to regain skills that might have been impacted. Physical
therapists might work with them to help them relearn coordination of their lower body movements to help them walk
again, or to learn how to get dressed using only one hand and
arm. Occupational therapists can also help transition the person to home, making recommendations for various adaptive
devices, for example, eating utensils with angled, foam han-
dles to facilitate eating and/or clothing with larger arm and
leg holes and/or velcro closures to help the person dress more
easily. A speech therapist may help your caregivee/loved one
relearn how to communicate effectively, and may be called
upon to make recommendations if the caregivee/loved one is
having swallowing difficulties.

Rehabilitation may start as early as 48 hours post-stroke
at an inpatient hospital. Skilled nursing facilities can also
provide skilled rehabilitation services. Home health agencies

provide services in the home and can often adapt to your caregivee/loved one's daily schedule. Home care services can be provided if the caregivee/loved one meets the criteria set by Medicare or your insurance company to receive care in the home. The doctor will work with your caregivee/loved one and other members of the rehabilitation team to establish the best treatment plan for your caregivee/loved one.

Upon returning home after a stroke, your caregivee/loved one may receive in-home rehabilitation. If this is the case, you may have a variety of health care providers coming to the home. This can be daunting—so many people to keep track of and all of them teaching new things, new medications, new techniques, new equipment. Help the home care team to help you by being ready for their visit. A calendar is useful to organize which team member is coming and when. Encourage the care team to write when their next visit will be on the calendar. By being prepared, the visits can be accomplished in the most efficient manner and you and your caregivee/loved one can return to your "new" normal life with new strategies tailored specifically for your caregivee/loved one's needs. After the initial "flurry" of activity, you and your caregivee/ loved one are sure to find a comfortable day-to-day routine. Hopefully, you will have identified (or been told!) who the best contact person is on the home care team and you should always call them if you have any questions or concerns.

3. General Goals for Care: Bottom line goals: Manage risk factors to prevent another stroke and help your caregivee/ loved one regain as much independence as possible after a stroke.

The symptoms of a stroke vary and much depends upon

the age of the person and the type of stroke. The National Institute of Health reports that 15 to 30 percent of stroke survivors will have a permanent physical disability (Know-Stroke, 2009). And unfortunately, 20 percent of people who have a first stroke between the ages of 40 and 69 will have another stroke within five years (KnowStroke, 2009). The risk of a stroke within 90 days of a TIA is 10 to 20 percent (KnowStroke, 2009). As a caregiver, you may find your role changing as your caregivee/loved one regains strength and independence. Sadly, their care needs may increase if new challenges arise.

The warning signs of a stroke should be recognized and addressed immediately. The person experiencing a stroke must get to a hospital quickly! Treatment begins immediately and is often designed to either dissolve the blood clot or stop the bleeding. It is optimal if the person can be treated within three hours of the first onset of symptoms. The symptoms of a stroke include, but are not limited to: sudden confusion; trouble speaking; trouble understanding speech; sudden trouble walking; dizziness; a change in balance or coordination; a sudden severe headache of unknown cause; sudden weakness; numbness; tingling of the face, arm, or leg, especially on one side of the body. The **FAST** test is a way to quickly assess if someone is having a stroke.

F: FACE	Ask the person to smile. Does one side of the face droop?
A: ARMS	Ask the person to raise both arms. Does one arm drift down?
S: SPEECH	Ask the person to repeat a simple sentence. Is the speech slurred or garbled?

T: TIME   If you observe any of these signs, either together or alone, call 911 immediately!

(The American Stroke Association, n.d.)

Check the time when you do this and tell the emergency responders and emergency department care team. This information is very valuable for them to know. Tell them if your caregivee/loved one has had a previous stroke.

Women may experience unique symptoms of stroke. These symptoms may appear suddenly and include, but are not limited to: hiccups, face or limb pain, shortness of breath, nausea, chest pain, and general weakness. If you see these symptoms, call 911.

For a recurrent stroke, be an assertive caregivee/loved one advocate and insist on an MRI or CAT scan for specific diagnosis information; CAT scan may be a better choice since they typically take less time than an MRI (NIHSenior-Health, n.d.).

If hypertension was a contributing factor to the person's stroke, they may be prescribed medication(s) to control it. These medications could include diuretics, often referred to as "water pills," to reduce the amount of fluid in the person's system; beta blockers to decrease heart rate; and/or calcium channel blockers to lower blood pressure and improve circulation. After a stroke, many people are prescribed "blood thinners" to prevent blood clots. These are only examples of medications that the doctor may prescribe, not an inclusive list or recommendation. Your caregivee/loved one will likely have a medication regimen tailored specifically for them. Always follow the doctors instructions regarding medications, and if you have any questions about the medications prescribed, speak with the doctor or pharmacist. If the doctor prescribed blood thinners for your caregivee/loved one, they may need regular blood tests to make sure the blood is not too thin, which could lead to bleeding, or too thick, which could lead to clotting. There are new medications that may not need this monitoring. Any new medications should be checked for interactions with anticoagulants before it is administered. This includes all herbal medications and over the counter products. It is important to keep all appointments for blood work. These test results should be given to the doctor so that changes can be made to the medication dosage as needed. Keeping a log/notebook, by writing on a calendar, is a good idea, and it is strongly encouraged. Write down any blood test appointments, results, and medication changes as well as any symptoms or changes your caregivee/loved one may have had on this calendar and have it handy if you call the doctor or nurse. Bring it and all medications, including over-the-counter medications, vitamins or supplements, and medications prescribed by other physicians with you to any doctor's appointments or emergency department visits.

You will want to watch for signs of bleeding. Signs of bleeding can include: bruises under the skin; bleeding gums; or black, sticky, tar-like stools. If you see any of these signs of bleeding, call the doctor, nurse, or health care team right away. Be especially cautious if your caregivee/loved one experiences a fall and monitor them closely for signs and symptoms of bleeding. Always call the doctor, nurse, or other health care team member and report that your caregivee/loved one fell, and be sure to tell them that the person takes blood thinners. Your caregivee/loved one may be on a blood thinner medication that does not require regular blood tests, and, if this is the case, please watch them very carefully for signs of bleeding as well.

Your caregivee/loved one may be taking a diuretic medication sometimes referred to as a "water pill" to remove excess fluid from the body. Diuretics are given to lower blood pressure and to reduce stress on the heart. This medication may cause a person to urinate more frequently. Diuretics are usually taken in the morning so that your caregivee/loved one can experience a good night's sleep. The fluid that your caregivee/loved one is eliminating does not need to be replaced. This medication may cause people to experience a dry mouth. If this is the case, sucking on hard candy or ice chips may alleviate dry mouth without adding unwanted fluid back into the body. Ask the doctor if you have any questions about this or other facets of your caregivee/loved one's care.

Assisting the caregivee/loved one to monitor their blood pressure and keeping a record of it on the log/notebook is a great way to watch for any changes and is a handy tool for physician communication. Again, bring their log/notebook with you (along with all of the medications) to any doctor's appointments. Have it handy as well when you call the doctor's office or speak with the nurse or any other members of the health care team. The doctor will tell you what their healthy blood pressure range is and how often you should take a blood pressure reading. If you have not been shown how to take a blood pressure reading, please ask to be shown! Some local grocery stores and pharmacies now have simple blood pressure stations that are designed for the public to use. Use them! You can also purchase simple battery operated blood pressure devices at most pharmacies or drug stores. If you see a higher or lower reading than normal, call the doctor, nurse, or health care team.

Other ways to help the person with high blood pressure include encouraging/helping them with lifestyle changes, such as: developing and maintaining healthy eating habits, losing weight (if recommended), quitting smoking, encouraging a daily or weekly exercise program, and taking all medications as prescribed. By controlling high blood pressure, you are also helping to control heart disease, diabetes, and kidney failure, all of which contribute to stroke risk. A healthy lifestyle is recommended because it affects all aspects of general health. As you have seen, all of our body systems are interwoven. This is very evident when discussing reducing stroke risk.

Cutting down on salt (or sodium) intake, eating less red meat, eating more fruits and vegetables, decreasing saturated fats in the diet contributes to good general health. Salt, or sodium, causes fluid to build up in the body, and this fluid buildup causes the heart to work harder. It can also cause arteries to thicken, again affecting the heart and contributing to both high blood pressure and stroke. Some salt in the diet is necessary, but in small amounts. Examples of high salt or high sodium foods are: canned soups, dry soup mixes, canned meats and fish, bacon, ham, sausage, butter, margarine, and packaged frozen dinners or other frozen food products. Only use salt substitutes if recommended by the doctor. Use low salt seasonings such as lemon juice and herbs. Fresh or frozen vegetables are always best, but canned fruits and vegetables are available that are "low-sodium."

Saturated fats can cause cholesterol levels to rise. Cholesterol is the waxy/fatty deposits, called "plaque" that can line the blood vessels and cause atherosclerosis. As we have seen, atherosclerosis is the enemy; it has been strongly linked to cardiac disease and stroke. Limiting red meats, butter, dairy products, eggs, shortening, lard, and palm and coconut oils in the diet will decrease the saturated fats in your diet. Any fat that is not liquid at room temperature is best avoided. Many fast foods are high in sodium *and* saturated fats. Those with diabetes should avoid food particularly high in sodium and processed sugar.

Drinks containing alcohol decrease the heart's ability to contract, and, again, this ultimately affects blood pressure. Drinks containing alcohol should be eliminated or limited to one drink, two to three times a week. "One drink" means a small glass of wine, beer or 1 ounce of alcohol in a mixed drink. Water and juice are always better choices.

The National Institutes of Health reports that cigarette smoking doubles the risk of ischemic stroke and quadruples the risk of hemorrhagic stroke (NINDS, 2014). It is linked to atherosclerosis of the carotid arteries, and blockage of a carotid artery is the leading cause of stroke (NINDS, 2014).

The nicotine in cigarettes raises blood pressure and the carbon monoxide in cigarette smoke reduces the amount of oxygen in the blood. Cigarette smoke thickens the blood and makes clotting more likely. And, if that isn't bad enough, cigarette smoke causes a weakening of the walls of the arteries (think: hemorrhagic stroke). If your caregivee/loved one is having trouble quitting smoking, please encourage them to speak with their doctor, nurse, or health care team. Smoking is a very difficult addiction to overcome, but recovery from cigarette smoking is possible. The doctor may prescribe medication or recommend a program that could make all the difference "this time." Quitting smoking often requires several attempts and "this time" may just be the right time. There are phone apps that measure and count the days, weeks, and/ or months since the last cigarette and display the number of cigarettes that would have been smoked and the money saved. These apps can provide added incentives to help a person stop smoking. The U.S. government has a website devoted to helping people quit smoking: http://smokefree.gov/

A physical exercise program for a person recovering from a stroke may be recommended once they have met the rehabilitation goals set for them. Recovery continues after a person's goals have been met and may include an exercise program developed with the person by the doctor and physical therapist. In general, a specialized exercise program has several benefits. It may lower weight and/or help maintain a healthy weight, and the CDC reports that exercise can lower cholesterol levels and blood pressure. Before starting any exercise program, always check with your doctor. As a general guideline, the CDC recommends two hours and thirty minutes of moderate to intense exercise per week as a way of preventing stroke (CDC, 2014). Your caregivee/loved one should approach any exercise training or physical activity program within the limits outlined for them by their physician. Talk with the physical therapist for recommendations about exercises that they can do at home.

4. Personal Care Considerations: Going home can be challenging for both the caregivee/loved one and the caregiver. Tasks learned at the rehabilitation center may be difficult to transfer once back at home. When the person tries to return to old activities, the deficits from the stroke may become more apparent. The person may experience a difficult, but hopefully temporary, adjustment period. Persons returning home to a healthy caregiver are more likely to become independent again. Encouragement in a safe environment is as important as early treatment for the stroke survivor.

Maintaining an open line of communication with your caregivee/loved one is vital. It allows you awareness of any physical and/or emotional changes. Anticipate that the caregivee/loved one may be "up and down" emotionally. This is called being emotionally labile. This can occur as a direct result of the stroke and/or as a response to the sudden change in lifestyle. Stroke survivors may be coping with unspoken fears that the stroke might happen again, that they may not be able to adjust to the deficits that they incurred, that they may be placed in a nursing home, that the caregiver won't be able to "handle" their increased care needs, or that they may be abandoned by family and friends. Anticipate that during an adjustment period your caregivee/loved one may experience and display fear, anger, anxiety, depression, and loss of self-esteem. Your caregivee/loved one may appreciate a visit with the rehab team's social worker or psychologist to gain insight and develop post-stroke coping strategies.

The stroke may impact your relationship by changing established boundaries. You may suddenly find yourself providing care that is both personal and intimate. It might help to know that you are not alone. Attending a local community support group may be of tremendous help. The doctor, nurse, or social worker may be good resources for this type of information. The American Stroke Association offers a resource page for caregivers taking care of someone who has had a stroke: http://www.strokeassociation .org/STROKEORG/LifeAfterStroke/ForFamilyCaregivers/

For-Stroke-Family-Caregivers_UCM_308560_SubHome
Page.jsp

Keeping your caregivee/loved one clean, safe, and comfortable will be a consistent goal of personal care. Personal care may include activities such as getting in and out of bed, bathing, dressing, grooming, meal preparation, and assistance with feeding. Stroke survivors need an orderly and consistent environment with enough stimulation to keep them engaged, yet not so much that they become overwhelmed. Always tell your caregivee/loved one what you are going to do before you do it and what you are doing as you do it. Allow the person to be as involved as possible in making care decisions.

Try to return to previous daily routines, remembering that those routines may still be possible, but may not look exactly the same as they used to. Due to the variety of challenges that arise from a stroke, seek direct practical guidance and advice from your caregivee/loved one's medical, nursing, and rehabilitation care team. Use the time that they are visiting the home to ask questions and ask for demonstrations. Ask if you can "demonstrate back" to them what you have been taught to make sure you understood it correctly.

When a person experiences paralysis, it can show up as weakness and be accompanied by rigidity of muscles and/or spasticity of muscles. Spasticity describes jerking, disorganized, and unexpected, sudden movements. Both upper and lower limbs can be affected and can make balance and coordination difficult. Post-stroke walking may be unsafe and even painful because of weakness and spasticity. The leg may be unable to bear weight or the knee joint may hyperextend. There may be a loss of sensation, poor balance, and/or poor coordination. Your caregivee/loved one may experience anxiety or fear at their increased risk of falling.

The physical therapist often targets the relearning of motor skills. Physical therapists may teach stretching, walking, strengthening, gait training, coordination of safe transfers, and range of motion exercises. They often teach exercises for strength training. The physical therapist may make recommendations for walking aids and teach the person how to use them. To help a person during mealtimes, the speech or occupational therapist may recommend aids such as plate guards, placemats that won't slip, or other adaptive devices. A larger discussion for caregivers on the topic of home modifications and adaptive equipment can be found later in this chapter under safety considerations. You can also refer to Chapter Six: Safety in the Home: The Most Frequent Health Care Setting of Choice!

Your caregivee/loved one may have aphasia (ah-faze-jah), which is a language impairment due to stroke. Aphasia is very broad in scope. An aphasic person may have difficulty using or comprehending words. Aphasia may make it difficult to talk, read, write, and/or understand what others are saying, and/or there may be difficulty with numbers and/or number calculations. A speech therapist may recommend exercises, games, or puzzles as aids to regain language and speech skills. They can often provide or describe simple communication devices, such as an alphabet board. The occupational therapist may be able to make recommendations for addressing aphasia as well. The right communication aid can greatly enhance communication. Keep trying until you find the right one.

The following tips might be helpful for communicating with

a person who is aphasic: Talk to the person as an adult, not a child. Do not talk down to an aphasic person, but keep your words to them simple and concise. Do not shout; stroke does not usually affect a person's hearing. Limit background noise, which can be distracting. Turn off televisions and radios when speaking. Have the person's attention before speaking and allow time for the caregivee/loved one to focus. Allow time for them to process what has been said. Make speaking a pleasurable experience, not a chore. Praise their attempts to converse. Use and encourage various types of communication, such as hand/finger tapping, eye movements, and eye contact. Be creative! Try writing or drawing to communicate. Avoid correcting the caregivee/loved one too frequently. Do not demand that words be pronounced perfectly. Repeat a statement back to clarify that you understand what they have said. Only speak for the person if you have their permission. Be with the caregivee/loved one as they try to communicate with others. Include the person in family discussions, decisions, and in social conversations. Keep them informed of daily family activities and news events, but limit small details.

Please be aware that the social impact of aphasia can be devastating. Aphasic stroke survivors can find themselves isolated and ignored. Friends and family may stop calling and may stop inviting them places because they find conversation too difficult. It is rare that aphasic persons are able to return to the lives they had prior to the stroke. The frustration, boredom, and loneliness that this can cause are high risk factors for serious depression and suicide. Work closely with the person's rehab care team to recreate, enhance, and maintain communication skills and notify the doctor if you see signs and symptoms of depression in your caregivee/loved one.

Consider how frustrating it would be if you could not speak and/or be understood.

After a stroke, some people experience cognition or thinking deficits. This could mean difficulty remembering things, difficulty comprehending things, lessened self-awareness, and/or an inability to learn new information or tasks. They may have lost the ability to problem-solve, understand, or make plans. A person with cognitive deficits may not be able to acknowledge the reality of their situation. They may forget that they have a paralyzed or weakened side. They may be impulsive even if in the past they were not. The cognitively impaired stroke survivor may have poor judgment and may need assistance making big decisions.

Such cognitive deficits can be difficult for the caregiver trying to manage daily tasks and personal care. Try breaking tasks up into simple steps, and establish a routine. Keep items that are used daily in the same place. Use keywords to prompt or remind your caregivee/loved one of the next step. Playing memory games, card games, and word games, such as crossword, may improve cognition in some people. Look to the person's speech or occupational therapist for resources.

If your caregivee/loved one is confined to bed, you will find the section "Bedbound Care (Care of the Immobilized or Bedridden Patient)" helpful. The biggest risk to bedbound people are bedsores, also called "pressure ulcers." Be sure to move your caregivee/loved one often to protect their skin. It is important that your caregivee/loved one's joints and muscles be maintained as functional as possible. If your caregivee/loved one has a paralyzed limb and sits or lies in one position for too long, this can cause the body to stiffen and cause an aching pain, especially in the joints. The goal is to keep the bones, joints, and muscles moving safely to preserve their ongoing ability to move. Practice range of motion exercises as recommended. If you have questions, the physical therapist can show you and your caregivee/loved one how to safely perform both active and passive range of motion exercises.

Some post-stroke caregivee/loved ones are unable to control their bladder and/or bowels. This is called "incontinence" and can be common in the time period just after a stroke. You may hear the term "voiding" used, which refers to urination. The doctor, nurse, or other health care team members may recommend "bladder training" to help your caregivee/loved one regain bladder control. You may be taught how to set up a voiding schedule. Bladder training is most successful if you stick to the schedule as much as possible. Physical exercises and deep breathing exercises may be recommended as well. Diet adjustments, such as not drinking liquids after a certain time of day, may help. In some cases, the doctor might prescribe medications or a urinary catheter. A bedside commode may be helpful. Ask your caregivee/loved one's health care team for recommendations. If your caregivee/loved one is incontinent, scrupulous skin care is a must. Skin care is addressed more specifically in the section "Bedbound Care (Care of the Immobilized or Bedridden Patient)" and incontinence is further addressed in "Urinary and Incontinence Care."

5. Safety Considerations: Stroke survivors may experience trouble swallowing. This is called dysphagia (dis-fah-gee-ah) and can be caused by paralysis or weakness of the mouth and/or throat. Swallowing difficulties can happen gradually over time. Always stay with your caregivee/loved one during meal times. A soft-food diet or pureed diet may be recommended by the speech therapist. Always pay close attention to your caregivee/loved one's breathing and swallowing during mealtimes. Choking can block the person's airway; if this happens, it is an emergency and you should call 911. A person with dysphagia can accidentally send food or liquid into their lungs. This will cause them to cough and coughing forcefully may help them to clear their lungs. If you notice any changes to your caregivee/loved one's ability to breathe or swallow, let the doctor, nurse, or other health care member know right away. Even a small amount of food or liquid sent to the caregivee/loved one's lungs, called "aspiration," can quickly develop into an infection and possibly pneumonia.

Be aware that if the person is fatigued, or for other reasons associated with stroke, they may "pocket" food on the side or toward the back of their mouth. Notify the health care team if you see this happening. Your caregivee/loved one may find it easier to swallow thickened liquids rather than thin liquids. Thickened liquids may be recommended by the doctor or the speech language pathologist, and the health care team can show you how to achieve this. Only provide food in the texture/consistency recommended by the doctor.

Helping your caregivee/loved one maintain a clean, fresh mouth is both a safety and a comfort measure. Attentive mouth care may prevent and help detect mouth problems early on. Stroke survivors may have a weakened immune system, which puts them at risk for mouth infections. Notify the doctor, nurse, or health care team if your caregivee/loved one develops any mouth sores, white spots, or a white coating on their tongue.

Home modifications may be necessary to allow a person

a greater level of independence and safety in the home. The nurse, physical therapist, occupational therapist, and social worker can offer you and your caregivee/loved one guidance regarding these adaptations. Modifications may include installing ramps, rearranging furniture, and/or removing furniture and rugs that could create fall hazards. Perhaps the person will need to stay on the ground floor or perhaps a chair lift could be installed. Modifications may also include lighting installations to ensure adequate lighting in walkways and stairwells. Install sturdy stair railings and add railings to hallways and stairs if needed. Doorways may need to be widened to accommodate a wheelchair. Installing "grab bars" in the bathroom and shower is an invaluable safety measure. Consider having a walker/assistive device on each floor/level of the home.

Other medical/safety equipment could include a "gait belt" to help transfer the person from sitting to standing and back again as well as to improve safety when walking. In addition, a cane, a walker, a wheelchair, a raised toilet seat, a shower chair, a hand-held shower head, and bed rails may also be helpful in supporting safety. Safety or body monitors allow you to hear someone in another room and walkie-talkies allow you to communicate from one part of the house to another. You may consider a chair or bed "monitor," which is a small electronic device that will alert you if your caregivee/loved one is at risk to fall, such as standing up to walk from a chair or bed. Members of the rehabilitation team can make these recommendations and show you which ones may be best suited for your caregivee/loved one. The team social worker may be able to help you and your caregivee/loved one with financial information and other resources for equipment.

Please consider emergency access should you be away from home. Perhaps install a lock box or leave a key with a neighbor. You may want to ask for recommendations from your local police or fire department. Doing this may prevent emergency personnel from having to knock down your door in the event of an emergency. Discuss this with your caregivee/loved one if an emergency alert device would be helpful.

Seizures are episodes of abnormal or disorganized electrical activity in the brain. Stroke is the most common cause of seizures in older adults (National Stroke Association, n.d.). Sometimes seizures can mimic a stroke. A person having a seizure may stare into space. They may convulse, meaning they have violent spasmodic muscle contractions.

If your caregivee/loved one is having a seizure, remain calm and protect them from harm and embarrassment. Roll them onto their side to prevent choking, in case they vomit. Do not put anything in their mouth. Do not give them liquids or medication during a seizure. Cushion their head and move them safely away from any sharp objects that could accidentally hurt them. Call 911 and stay with your caregivee/loved one until the seizure ends and 911 arrives.

Note how long the seizure lasts and what the symptoms were, and give this information to the emergency responders. If your caregivee/loved one experiences recurrent seizures, their doctor may prescribe medication. Please be aware that missing a dose of this medication, not getting enough sleep, and drinking alcohol are all factors that can contribute to seizures. Seizures can be distressing and embarrassing for your caregivee/loved one; they often lose control of their bladder during a seizure. Protect their privacy and dignity at all times.

6. When to Call the Doctor, Nurse, or Care Team: These are only possible examples and NOT an inclusive list. Please remember that calling *before* a situation becomes a bigger problem is always best. It's better to catch problems when they are relatively small. It is much harder to address "big" problems.

- Caregivee/loved one has facial drooping.
- Caregivee/loved one has one-sided weakness.
- Caregivee/loved one cannot repeat a simple sentence and/or they have slurred or garbled speech.
- Caregivee/loved one has difficulty swallowing or changes to their swallowing.
- Caregivee/loved one has a change in how they urinate. Perhaps they cannot urinate or they are urinating much more frequently than usual, but only producing small amounts of urine. Perhaps their urine has changed color, is very dark, and/or has a strong odor.
- Caregivee/loved one has had a change in their bowel movements or has stopped having bowel movements for more than three days, even if they are not eating very much.
- Caregivee/loved one has fallen.
- Caregivee/loved one has an area of redness on their skin that does not go away shortly after repositioning them.
- Caregivee/loved one has unexplained bruising, or tiny red dots on the skin.
- Caregivee/loved one has unexplained bleeding from gums or nose.
- Caregivee/loved one has bright red vomit or vomit that looks like coffee grounds.
- Caregivee/loved one has blood in their urine or stools or has black, tarry stools.

- Caregivee/loved one experiences a loss of feeling or a loss of movement in one of their limbs.
- Caregivee/loved one has sudden, severe head pain, chest pain, or abdominal pain.
- Caregivee/loved one has a sudden or high fever.
- Caregivee/loved one shows a personality change and/or has an increase in confusion.
- Caregivee/loved one cannot get comfortable or find relief from pain. For example, pain wakes caregivee/loved one up at night or pain comes on suddenly.
- Caregivee/loved one has white spots or a white coating on their tongue, or any other kind of mouth sore. This may or may not be accompanied by difficulty swallowing.
- Caregivee/loved one is very emotional, perhaps they cannot stop crying or they are showing other obvious signs of emotional distress.
- Caregivee/loved one is questioning their spiritual beliefs, perhaps doubting what they once believed.
- Caregivee/loved one has other signs or symptoms of depression.
- Any other change, complication, or concern that you or the caregivee/loved one may have. When in doubt, call!

These are examples only. Your caregivee/loved one might relay to you changes or concerns that vary from those listed here and those concerns should be addressed with your care team.

7. Comfort Considerations: Comfort for your caregivee/ loved one can mean physical, mental, spiritual, or any combination of these things. Anticipating the comfort needs of a person following a stroke may feel daunting or overwhelming to both the person and caregiver, especially when they first return home.

As a caregiver, providing comfort for your caregivee/loved one sometimes means "the small things." Small things are sometimes easily overlooked. Having regular bowel movements may seem like a small thing, but it is actually a very large part of comfort. If the person's stroke involved their lower body, bowel movements can be a concern. They may experience incontinence and/or constipation. The doctor or nurse can make recommendations for incontinence care or other products or treatment to address these issues, such as stool softeners.

If your caregivee/loved one is on any pain medication, they can and, in many cases, do cause constipation. It is always better to prevent a problem than to correct a problem in regards to bowel movements. This is especially true with pain medications and constipation. We encourage you not to be shy about discussing bowel habits with your caregivee/loved one. Contact the doctor or nurse if their bowels have not moved for three days. This is true even if they are not eating very much. Bowel movements are something that should be tracked in the log/notebook.

Bringing stroke survivors on grocery store trips can keep them involved and may "normalize" their post-stroke lifestyle. It can help keep them involved in family activities and allows them to participate in their meal selections. Mall walking and exercise videos are other possible healthy distractions. Ask the rehab team for resources for chair yoga, chair stretching and chair exercises. Be creative, adapt as needed, persevere, and try to remain positive and inclusive. Healthy outcomes and recovery are possible!

If you are planning an outing for your caregivee/loved one, set yourself up for success by being proactive. Think through the outing before you go. Plan it for a time of day that the person has the most energy, perhaps in the morning. Consider the amount of time the activity will take and gauge their stamina level to ensure success. A half-day outing may be the best plan. Perhaps visit the location first to check accessibility. Consider the distance to the planned outing. Is the person fatigued after a long car ride? If the person has one-sided weakness, consider logistics, such as parking and the locations and size of the rest rooms. Consider the amount of time the activity will take. Remember that stimulation such as loud music, background noise, and crowds can overwhelm a stroke survivor in a short period of time and plan accordingly. Plan rest periods and bring medications along. Perhaps bring energy-packed snacks to help fight fatigue. Invite a friend along for added support.

Your caregivee/loved one may experience difficulty sleeping at night. Insomnia may have a negative impact on stroke recovery and can disrupt the caregiver's sleep patterns as well. Naps during the daytime may help if your caregivee/loved one is feeling tired from lack of sleep. Notify the doctor if they experience shortness of breath and/or coughing when they lie flat. Lying flat may cause difficulty breathing for some persons post-stroke. Using more than one pillow to prop up the head and upper body may help. Keeping the head and chest elevated by raising the mattress from underneath may be comforting. The doctor, nurse, or other rehab team member may suggest purchasing a foam "wedge" pillow to lay on or to position under the mattress to facilitate breathing. A reclining chair can also be considered. Sleep disruption may be caused by anxiety. If anxiety is not well addressed with non-pharmaceutical measures, speak with the doctor. An anti-anxiety or sleep medication may be prescribed. As with any medication, monitor the caregivee/loved one for changes and prevent falls where possible.

Spending time with a beloved pet is often wonderful therapy for those who are feeling "down" or depressed. Distractions, such as watching a movie or playing a game, may help address the anxiety or depression that some post-stroke caregivee/loved ones experience. If your caregivee/loved one is spiritually inclined, but not very mobile, a home visit from their clergy member or a chaplain may be helpful. A chaplain may be a member of the rehab team. As always, communicate with your caregivee/loved one and ask them to guide you specifically to best address their unique needs.

Sometimes your caregivee/loved one may ask to be left alone for a while. Please don't take this personally. A stroke can be devastating. It affects not just the person, but those around them as well, perhaps most especially, the caregiver. Persons who have had a stroke can feel anxious, depressed, and sometimes grouchy. Give your caregivee/loved one "alone time" if they need it, and, if possible, use this time to do something nice for yourself. If your caregivee/loved one doesn't recover from their need to be alone after a day or two, they may be experiencing depression. Talk with them about it.

The caregivee/loved one's depression can also affect the caregiver. It may make you feel unappreciated or less enthusiastic about providing care. It can make other family members or friends feel less inclined to visit or socialize with the stroke survivor. For these reasons, it may be time to call the doctor, nurse, social worker, or other rehab care team member. Post-stroke depression might be treated with individual or group therapy and/or medication. There are many antidepressant medications. If one is prescribed and you see little or no improvement after the timeframe specified, speak with the doctor. A different medication may be a better medication to meet your particular caregivee/loved one's needs.

In regard to discomfort or pain, changing positions, a gentle back rub, or a massage may help ease pain. A heating pad or cold/ice compress often helps with pain. Be sure to ask the doctor, nurse, or health care team before using any heat or cold on any person who has mobility issues or decreased sensation/numbness. Always protect their skin by placing a cloth between their skin and the source of heat or cold. Replace any heating pad that has a frayed cord and be very careful with heating pads. Immobile caregivee/loved ones have very fragile skin. Heat packs that are heated in a micro-wave oven are not recommended.

Believe your caregivee/loved one if they indicate to you that they have pain. Paralysis and weakness does not mean that a post-stroke caregivee/loved one cannot feel pain. Let the doctor know that your caregivee/loved one is having pain and follow any medication instructions carefully. Monitor closely for constipation. If the pain medication prescribed does not ease the caregivee/loved one's pain, let the doctor know. No person should ever be left in pain.

8. Special Considerations: Respite care is a type of short-term care provided to the person that allows the caregiver a break from caregiving activities. Respite care may be an op-tion for you, the caregiver. The person's nurse or social worker may be good resources of information for you regarding respite care. Not all insurance programs cover respite care, but some do. You may find information at the federal government website for the Administration on Aging (www.aoa.gov) and/or your state government's agency on aging. When choosing a respite care provider, discuss payment in advance, conduct background checks if possible, check work and personal references, and always interview the respite providers before engaging them.

9. Special Instructions Given to You by the Doctor, Nurse, or Care Team:

_____

_____

_____

_____

_____

_____

_____

_____

_____

10. Resources:

- The National Institute of Neurological Disorders and Stroke (NINDS) offers a "Post-Stroke Rehabilitation Fact Sheet": http://www.ninds.nih.gov/disorders/stroke/post strokerehab.htm
- NIHSeniorHealth offers information about stroke including prevalence and the differences between hemorrhagic and ischemic strokes: http://nihseniorhealth.gov/stroke/aboutstroke/01.html

- The American Stroke Association offers information about transient ischemic attacks (TIAs): http://www.stroke association.org/STROKEORG/AboutStroke/Typesof Stroke/TIA/TIA-Transient-Ischemic-Attack_UCM_ 310942_Article.jsp
- Mass.gov offers resources about stroke, including some in Spanish, Portuguese, and Khmer, on their website: http:// www.mass.gov/eohhs/gov/departments/dph/programs/ community-health/heart-disease-stroke/
- The American Speech-Language-Hearing Association has resources if your patient is experiencing trouble speaking: http://www.asha.org/
- A good book to help caregivers, friends, and family members understand what it is like to have a stroke is *My Stroke of Insight: A Brain Scientist's Personal Journey* by Jill Bolte Taylor.

References

Centers for Disease Control and Prevention (CDC). (2013). Cerebrovascular Disease or Stroke. Retrieved from http://www.cdc.gov/nchs/fastats/stroke.htm

Centers for Disease Control and Prevention (CDC). (2014). Preventing Stroke: Healthy Living. Retrieved from http://www.cdc.gov/stroke/healthy_living.htm

Harvard School of Public Health Nutrition Source. (n.d.). Fats and Cholesterol. Retrieved from http://www.hsph.harvard.edu/nutritionsource/what-should-you-eat/fats-and-cholesterol/

Kratz, M. (2005). Dietary cholesterol, atherosclerosis and coronary heart disease. *Handbook of Experimental Pharmacology*, (170):195–213.

KnowStroke. (2009). Stroke: Challenges, Progress, and Promise. Retrieved from http://stroke.nih.gov/materials/strokechallenges.htm

National Institute of Neurological Disorders and Stroke (NINDS). (2013).

What You Need to Know About Stroke. Retrieved from http://www .ninds.nih.gov/disorders/stroke/stroke_needtoknow.htm

National Institute of Neurological Disorders and Stroke (NINDS). (2014). Brain Basics: Preventing Stroke. Retrieved from http://www.ninds.nih .gov/disorders/stroke/preventing_stroke.htm

National Stroke Association. (n.d.). Seizures and Epilepsy. Retrieved from http://www.stroke.org/we-can-help/survivors/stroke-recovery/ post-stroke-conditions/physical/seizures-and-epilepsy

NIHSeniorHealth. (n.d.). Stroke. Retrieved from http://nihseniorhealth .gov/stroke/preventionanddiagnosis/01.html

The American Stroke Association. (2012). Stroke Risk Factors. Retrieved from http://www.strokeassociation.org/STROKEORG/AboutStroke/ UnderstandingRisk/Understanding-Stroke-Risk_UCM_308539_ SubHomePage.jsp

The American Stroke Association. (n.d.). Spot a Stroke. Retrieved from http://www.strokeassociation.org/STROKEORG/WarningSigns/ Stroke-Warning-Signs-and-Symptoms_UCM_308528_SubHomePage .jsp

URINARY AND INCONTINENCE CARE

1. Introduction: Incontinence or the accidental leakage of urine or stool can happen for a variety of reasons. Incontinence can happen to both men and women, but according to the National Kidney and Urologic Diseases Information Clearinghouse (NKUDIC), women experience urinary incontinence twice as often as men (2013). Incontinence can be either a temporary or a persistent problem.

Alcohol, caffeine, drinking too much fluid, foods with high sugar content, constipation, or a urinary tract infection can all cause temporary incontinence. Once the underlying cause is addressed, the incontinence problem may resolve.

Persistent incontinence can be caused by various physical changes that can include aging, an enlarged prostate, an obstruction within the urinary tract, various cancers, and neuromuscular disorders, such as Parkinson's disease or multiple sclerosis (MS).

A person may also have a urinary catheter. A urinary catheter is a tube that drains urine away from the body into a collection bag. A urinary catheter may be used because of urinary retention, possibly due to bladder atony, which means the person is unable to urinate; they may have had surgery that makes a catheter necessary; or another health problem, such as a spinal cord injury, could be the cause. Treatments for urinary incontinence depend upon its cause and severity.

2. General Information: If incontinence is a new occurrence for your caregivee/loved one, let the doctor, nurse, or health care team know as soon as possible. A urinary tract infection (UTI) may be the cause of sudden or new incontinence and this will need to be treated as soon as possible. In fact, in older adults, a UTI can cause confusion, falls, or other problems and so it needs to be treated right away.

Sleeping pills or anti-anxiety medications can sometimes be the cause of urinary incontinence. Caffeine in coffee, tea, and cola can increase urination urgency and frequency. You may want to limit fluids after a certain time of day to help prevent overnight incontinence, or the need to get up at night. However, do not withhold fluids to prevent incontinence in general because this can actually contribute to a UTI. Always ask the doctor if you have any questions about your caregivee/loved one's fluid intake, especially if they have "fluid restrictions" as part of their treatment plan.

Incontinence products may be helpful. There are many different types available, both disposable and non-disposable. There are products designed specifically for men and for women and there are products for daytime use and for overnight use. Look for pads or adult incontinence briefs that are absorbent and that present a quick-drying surface to protect the skin. Your caregivee/loved one may need to try a few different kinds or brands until they find "the right fit." Most drug stores and big box stores carry these products. Ask your doctor, nurse, or health care team to recommend a product suitable for your particular caregivee/loved one's needs. Consider, too, other incontinence products, such as waterproof mattress covers and incontinence pads for the bed and to protect furniture.

Some people with persistent incontinence may have a urinary drainage system commonly referred to as a "urinary catheter with a bag." This device drains urine from the body, into the bag. Your caregivee/loved one may have an indwelling urinary catheter, a condom type urinary catheter, or a "suprapubic" urinary catheter. "Catheter" refers to the tubing that is connected to the bag that collects the urine. The catheter may be made of latex, silicone, or other synthetic material. Urinary drainage systems work by using gravity to drain urine into the bag. This bag should always remain lower than their waist and should never be placed on the floor for infection control reasons. The urine collection bags can be "leg bags," which are attached to the lower leg, usually with velcro straps, and can be worn under clothing, or "overnight bags," which are larger and appropriate for overnight use.

An indwelling urinary catheter drainage system consists of a sterile catheter placed into the caregivee/loved one's bladder through the urethra. The urethra is the opening in the body where urine comes out. The catheter is held in place or "anchored" in the bladder by a small, inflated balloon. This tubing is then connected to the drainage bag. You may hear this type of urinary drainage system referred to as a "Foley catheter."

A person with an indwelling urinary catheter should never pull or tug at it or try to remove it on their own. The doctor will determine how long the indwelling urinary catheter will stay in place or how often it needs to be changed. Placing an indwelling urinary catheter is a sterile procedure usually performed by a nurse or doctor. To remove the catheter, the nurse or doctor deflates the balloon and gently slides the catheter out.

An indwelling urinary catheter can be for short-term or long-term use. When a person has an indwelling urinary catheter, they may be more at risk for an infection of the urinary tract or kidneys (MedlinePlus, n.d.a). Sometimes these infections, called "catheter-associated urinary tract infections" or CAUTIs, can be resistant to antibiotics. Always watch for signs and symptoms of a UTI in a person with an indwelling urinary catheter. Be alert for a sudden fever, new or increased confusion, a change in urine color, blood in the urine, or a change in urine odor.

A condom catheter is a urinary drainage system for men. It sounds like what it is. It is worn on the outside of the penis and it looks very similar to a condom, but with a tube attached on the tip that allows urine to drain into a collection bag. Condom catheters are often used for male caregivee/ loved ones who are confused or who have dementia and may be at risk for tugging at or pulling out an indwelling catheter. The doctor, nurse, or other health care team member will recommend how often a condom catheter should be changed. Always inspect the skin of the penis for any redness, sores, or abrasions. If you have any concerns, contact your doctor before applying a new condom catheter. Condom catheters work best if they are applied to a clean, dry penis.

A "suprapubic" catheter is a urinary catheter inserted into the bladder through a small hole cut into the abdomen (belly). These catheters are usually changed every four to six weeks. Again, it depends upon the person's individual situation and the doctor's goal for care. Changing them requires "sterile technique" and is usually taught to you and/or your caregivee/loved one by the doctor, nurse, or other member of the health care team. If your caregivee/loved one has a suprapubic urinary catheter, you may be provided with a prescription from the doctor to purchase special catheters. You may also be given information about where to purchase them. If you have any questions about this, be sure to ask!

A person with a suprapubic catheter should check the catheter insertion site several times a day. The area around the catheter should be washed with mild soap and water every day. Pat it dry gently. Do not use creams or powders near the site. Your doctor, nurse, or other health care team member will show you how to apply bandages around the site. Always contact them if you have questions. As with any urinary catheter, keep the drainage bag below the waist, and off the floor. Try not to disconnect the tubing from the bag—this will keep the urine flowing better. Check for kinks and gently move the tubing around if it is not draining.

A person with a suprapubic catheter has slightly different care needs than a person with an indwelling or condom catheter. They are often advised to drink plenty of fluids, eight to 12 glasses of water every day for a few days after the catheter is changed, and to avoid strenuous exercise for one to two weeks after the catheter is changed. A person with a suprapubic catheter is sometimes advised to keep the catheter taped to the belly. Ask your doctor, nurse, or health care team for specific instructions or if you have any concerns. Use the following information provided by the National Institute of Health to help guide you:

MedlinePlus provides the following list for when to call the doctor or nurse:

- "You are having trouble changing your catheter or emptying your bag.
- "Your bag is filling up quickly, and you have an increase in urine.

- "You are leaking urine.
- "You notice blood in your urine a few days after you leave the hospital.
- "You are bleeding at the insertion site after you change your catheter, and it doesn't stop within 24 hours.
- "Your catheter seems blocked.
- "You notice grit or stones in your urine.
- "Your supplies do not seem to be working (balloon is not inflating or other problems).
- "You notice a smell or change in color in your urine, or your urine is cloudy.
- "You have signs of infection (a burning sensation when you urinate, fever, or chills)."

(MedlinePlus, n.d.b)

These are examples only. Your caregivee/loved one who has a suprapubic catheter might relay to you changes or concerns that vary from those listed here, and those considerations should be addressed with your care team.

If your caregivee/loved one has any type of urinary catheter, you will want to monitor that it is working properly (draining urine) and that the skin around the insertion sight is clean and free from any type of infection. Your caregivee/loved one should drink plenty of fluids during the day to keep the system working properly. Check that the tubing is not kinked if you see a decrease in urine flow. Urine should be "straw yellow" in color as a general rule, but ask the doctor what the right urine color is for your caregivee/loved one (Medline-Plus, n.d.c).

Medications and other factors, including some foods, can influence urine color and odor as well. For all catheters, try to avoid disconnecting the tubing from the bag, doing this can increase the risk of infection and might cause an "air lock" that can disrupt the urine flow. If you do disconnect or change the bags, wipe the end of the catheter tube gently with an alcohol wipe before reconnecting it to the bag. If any catheter becomes painful, clogged, or infected call the doctor, nurse, or health care team right away. Ask the nurse or health care team for recommendations on how to keep urinary drainage system bags clean.

3. General Goals for Care: Bottom line goals: prevent skin breakdown and monitor closely for a urinary tract infection.

When left on the skin, urine (and stool) quickly contributes to skin "breakdown," especially in persons who have limited mobility. Meticulous skin care is important to maintain skin that is free of reddened areas. Reddened areas can quickly become open wounds. Address soiling or a bowel movement immediately, as soon as possible, by changing any soiled undergarments and/or bed linen. Cleanse skin with mild soap and water, rinse and gently pat, do not rub, the skin dry. Your doctor, nurse, or health care team may recommend the use of "baby wipes" or other disposable products, and they may recommend products that do not contain alcohol. They may direct you to use a special skin lotion that protects the skin, sometimes called a "barrier cream." This would be applied to clean dry skin. Contact them before using any product on the caregivee/loved one's skin.

When moisture/soiling is persistent, you may be directed to use a special mattress, such as one made of dense foam, to help prevent pressure areas/skin break down. This type of mattress may provide extra comfort to your caregivee/loved one. These special mattresses or foam pads are also available for wheelchairs and may be recommended if they sit a lot. Encourage and/or assist your caregivee/loved one to change their position frequently to help prevent pressure sores. You will find useful information for preventing skin breakdown in the "Bedbound Care (Care of the Immobilized or Bedridden Patient)" section of this book.

Always be on the lookout for a UTI and, remember, a UTI can happen with or without a urinary catheter. Call the doctor, nurse, or health care team right away if you suspect a UTI. Signs of a UTI can be: increased confusion, restlessness, fever, decreased urine output, blood tinged urine, red and/or cloudy urine, urine with a strong odor or a new or unusual odor, pain at the insertion site, pain located around the lower back and sides, fever, tiredness or "shakiness," an urge to urinate (even with a catheter), pressure in the lower belly, and/or a burning sensation. Watch for non-verbal cues from your caregivee/loved one as well, such as pulling at clothing or restlessness. These are only some of the signs of a UTI. Your caregivee/loved one may "just not feel good" and, if this is the case, call. Always let the doctor, nurse, or other health care team member know that your caregivee/loved one has a urinary catheter. Unfortunately, sometimes they forget!

The following information provides a general guideline for caregivers caring for a person who has a urinary catheter. Involve your caregivee/loved one as much as possible in their daily care. Help them to stay aware of the position of the catheter and urine flow. It is best if your caregivee/loved one drinks more water than any other beverage and limits their caffeine intake. Encourage drinking fluids consistently throughout the day, every day. Increase fluid intake in hot weather. Paying attention to the color of the urine is a quick way to know if your caregivee/loved one is drinking enough. Notice changes: if the urine color is different, what might be the cause? Has your caregivee/loved one had less water or increased the number of caffeine drinks in the last 24 hours? Has a new medication been added, or a medication removed? Notice the flow of urine in the catheter after a position change and reposition it if needed.

4. Personal Care Considerations: As always, tell the person what you are going to do before you do it and what you are doing as you do it.

If your caregivee/loved one is incontinent, try not to embarrass them, and respect their need for privacy as much as possible. If appropriate, perhaps remind them to use the bathroom just before their usual time if you have noticed a pattern, for example, every two hours during the day. Providing reminders for a person, using adult language, and keeping the pathway to the bathroom well lit and free of clutter may help reduce incontinence.

Clothing that is easy to remove and easy to wash will be helpful for both you and your caregivee/loved one. Allow them plenty of time to urinate or move their bowels when they are in the bathroom, providing privacy if it is safe to do so. Sometimes, running water in the sink or dipping a hand into cool water can prompt a person to urinate.

If you are assisting a person who has a urinary catheter with bathing, use warm, soapy water and start where the catheter tube exits the body and wipe gently away from the person. Do not pull or tug on the catheter. Then rinse and dry, always washing, rinsing, and drying starting at the top and working away from the person. To prevent infection, always use a separate washcloth and towel from the one that is used to wash your caregivee/loved one. If the washcloth becomes soiled, use a new one. And, of course, as always, wear gloves and wash your hands before and after providing any personal care.

If your caregivee/loved one has a condom catheter, you may be instructed on how to apply it and how often it should be changed. Condom catheters work best if applied to a clean, dry penis. The doctor or nurse may recommend trimming pubic hair for cleanliness, caregivee/loved one comfort, and to help the condom adhere. Inspect the penis at every catheter change and report any redness or open areas to the doctor, nurse, or other health care team member right away. Do not apply a new condom catheter until instructed to do so by the doctor or nurse.

Always keep the drainage bag lower than the person's waist. Do not put it on the bed with the caregivee/loved one, for example, because this could cause the urine to flow back into the person. Keep the bag low so that gravity draws the urine away from the person and into the bag. Keep the tubing free from kinks, which might hinder the urine flow. Keep the bag off of the floor; hang it on the chair or bed lower than the person's waist using the hook provided. If it must be placed on the floor, place it on a clean surface, such as on a disposable incontinence sheet or in a container that can be easily cleaned, such as a dish pan, used only for this purpose. Empty the bag several times a day, as directed by the health care team.

If your caregivee/loved one has any type of urinary catheter, you will have been shown how to maintain it properly and how to empty the bag. If this has not been shown to you, please ask! Always wash your hands before and after providing any catheter care to prevent infection.

The doctor may ask you to keep a record of how much fluid your caregivee/loved one drinks in a day and/or the amount of urine output collected in a day. You may hear this referred to as "intake and output" or "I and O." Writing this information on a caregivee/loved one log or journal, perhaps using a calendar, can be a benefit to you, the caregivee/loved one, and their care team. Information such as when the catheter was first inserted or applied, when it needs to be changed, the start of any symptoms you may see, such as cloudy urine, the person's temperature, and the date that any medication was started are all examples of information to write in the care log. You may find it helpful to record bowel movements here as well. Bring this with you (with any and all medications!) when you take your caregivee/loved one to any doctor's appointments and have it handy if you need to call the doctor.

If your caregivee/loved one is incontinent of stool, be sure to wipe from front to back, keeping fecal matter away from the urethra and any catheter tubing. Use disposable wash cloths (ones without alcohol may be recommended) and never use a soiled washcloth or towel twice. If the washcloth becomes soiled, start fresh with a new one to prevent infection. Always wipe soiled areas away from where the catheter enters the body.

Studies are inconclusive regarding drinking cranberry juice and UTIs (Raz et al., 2004). It has been suggested that cranberry juice can "change" the lining of the urinary tract and may prevent organisms that cause UTI's from attaching or growing there. Ask the doctor if drinking cranberry juice or if taking cranberry tablets would benefit your caregivee/loved one, or if taking a cranberry supplement might also help (these have less sugar than drinking cranberry juice).

Sometimes people may feel embarrassed to be out in public, or even at home, if their urine drainage bag is visible, or if urine odor is detectable. A decorative, washable drawstring fabric "pouch" can be sewn and slipped over the bag for caregivee/loved one privacy. Incontinence can be very embarrassing for a person and it can strongly impact their personal sense of dignity. Respect their privacy and dignity at all times. There are "belly bags" for people who want to wear shorts and/or skirts.

5. Safety Considerations: Be cautious when assisting the person with repositioning, walking, and/or with personal care; be aware of where the tubing and bag is at all times to ensure that the tubing does not pull or kink or otherwise cause or contribute to a fall. Keep the tubing secured to the person's thigh as instructed by the nurse or health care team. They may provide you with a strap to secure the tubing to the thigh. If they have not done this, ask! Ask them to show you how to secure the tubing to the person's thigh to prevent accidently pulling on the tubing. Replace this strap if it becomes worn or soiled. Check the skin under the strap for redness, readjust it as needed, and be sure that it is not too tight.

A confused person may try to pull out an indwelling catheter and this could harm them. Call the doctor, nurse, or health care team right away if this happens! And remember that new or increased confusion can be a sign of a urinary tract infection so call the doctor, nurse, or health care team right away if you have concerns.

6. When to Call the Doctor, Nurse, or Care Team:

- Caregivee/loved one has bladder spasms—contractions of the bladder that cause urine to come out, sometimes accompanied by pain, that do not go away.
- Caregivee/loved one has bleeding into or around the catheter tubing.
- Caregivee/loved one has urine leaking onto the outside of the catheter tubing.
- Caregivee/loved one has very little or no urine in the tubing or bag.
- Caregivee/loved one has stones or sediment in the tubing or bag.
- Caregivee/loved one has swelling or sores around the area where the catheter inserts into the body (the urethra).
- Caregivee/loved one has increased confusion, restlessness, or is "pulling," for example, at clothing or sheets.
- Caregivee/loved one has a sudden or high fever.
- Caregivee/loved one has a change in how they urinate. Perhaps they cannot urinate or they are urinating much more frequently than usual, but only producing small amounts of urine. Perhaps their urine has changed color, is very dark, and/or has a strong odor.
- Caregivee/loved one has had a change in their bowel movements or has stopped having bowel movements for more than three days, even if they are not eating very much.
- Caregivee/loved one complains of pain.
- Caregivee/loved one has fallen.
- Any other change, complication, or concern that you or the caregivee/loved one may have. When in doubt, call!

These are examples only. Your caregivee/loved one might relay to you changes or concerns that vary from those listed here and those concerns should be addressed with your care team.

7. Comfort Considerations: Comfort for your caregivee/loved one can mean physical, mental, spiritual, or any combination of those kinds of comfort. As a caregiver, providing comfort for your caregivee/loved one sometimes means "the small things." Small things are sometimes easily overlooked. Having regular bowel movements may seem like a small thing, but it is actually a very large part of comfort. You may need to keep track of their bowel movements to identify and/or prevent constipation. If your caregivee/loved one is on any pain medication, they can and, in many cases, do cause constipation.

Constipation can cause pressure on the bladder and contribute to incontinence. It is a good idea to monitor bowel movements by recording them in their log/notebook. Contact the doctor, nurse, or health care team if your caregivee/loved one does not have a bowel movement for three days. This is true even if the caregivee/loved one is not eating very much. The doctor may suggest a stool softener or other medication.

8. Special Considerations: Persons with Alzheimer's disease may develop incontinence because they do not recognize the need to urinate or move their bowels or they may forget the location of the bathroom. Perhaps their clothing is too tight or they are confused as to how to remove clothing. Persons with Alzheimer's disease can develop a fear of water, and this may be the reason that they avoid the bathroom. A bedside commode or urinal (for a male caregivee/loved one) may be helpful in this case.

A person with Alzheimer's disease may have a "trigger" word that indicates that they need to go to the toilet. For example they may say "I need to talk to Mary" and, to them, those words mean "I need to go to the bathroom." Actively listen to your caregivee/loved one to identify their trigger words.

You may want to make the bathroom especially visible by leaving the light on or putting up a brightly colored poster where they can see it from outside the room. You may like to use glow-in-the dark tape to help them find their way. Perhaps remove objects that could be mistaken for a toilet, such as house plants, open waste baskets, spittoons, or other objects.

9. Special Instructions Given to You by the Doctor, Nurse, or Care Team:

_____

_____

_____

_____

_____

_____

_____

_____

10. Resources:

- National Kidney and Urologic Diseases Information Clearinghouse (NKUDIC) offers a page called "Urinary Incontinence in Women" that describes the prevalence of urinary incontinence and the reasons it is more common in women: http://kidney.niddk.nih.gov/KUDISEASES/pubs/uiwomen/index.aspx

- The NKUDIC also offers a resource called "The Urinary Tract and How It Works" to help you better understand what organs are part of the urinary tract and what they do: http://kidney.niddk.nih.gov/KUDiseases/pubs/yoururinary/

- Medline Plus also offers a diagram of the male urinary tract: http://www.nlm.nih.gov/medlineplus/ency/image pages/1123.htm

- There is also a diagram for the female urinary tract: http://www.nlm.nih.gov/medlineplus/ency/imagepages/1122.htm

- MedlinePlus has an explanation of urinary catheters as well: http://www.nlm.nih.gov/medlineplus/ency/article/003981.htm

- The Centers for Disease Control and Prevention (CDC) provide information on their site about "Catheter-associated Urinary Tract Infections" including treatment options for CAUTIs and prevention strategies: http://www.cdc.gov/HAI/ca_uti/cauti_faqs.html

- To learn more about suprapubic catheters in particular, visit Medline Plus's page on them: http://www.nlm.nih.gov/medlineplus/ency/patient oneinstructions/000145.htm

- The Louis Calder Memorial Library from the University of Miami Health System offers a resource called "Urinary Tract Management in Spinal Cord Injury: Urination and

the Urinary Tract in SCI: Indwelling Catheter": http://
calder.med.miami.edu/pointis/indwelling.html
- The Memorial Sloan Kettering Cancer Center has a
  caregivee/loved one education page called "Caring
  for Your Urinary (Foley) Catheter": http://www.mskcc
  .org/cancer-care/patient-education/resources/caring-your-
  urinary-foley-catheter
- AgingCare.com offers a guide for "The 4 Kinds of Urinary
  Incontinence": http://www.agingcare.com/Articles/types-of-
  urinary-incontinence-144709.htm

References

Medline Plus. (n.d.a). Catheter-related UTI. Retrieved from http://www
.nlm.nih.gov/medlineplus/ency/article/000483.htm

Medline Plus. (n.d.b). Suprapubic catheter care. Retrieved from http://
www.nlm.nih.gov/medlineplus/ency/patientinstructions/
000145.htm

MedlinePlus. (n.d.c). Urine—abnormal color. Retrieved from http://www
.nlm.nih.gov/medlineplus/ency/article/003139.htm

National Kidney and Urologic Diseases Information Clearinghouse
(NKUDIC). (2013). Urinary Incontinence in Women. Retrieved from
http://kidney.niddk.nih.gov/KUDISEASES/pubs/uiwomen/index.aspx

Raz, R, Chazan, B, Dan, M. (2004). Cranberry juice and urinary tract
infection. *Clinical Infectious Diseases.* 15;38(10):1413–9.

Index

NOTES

Date	Description

NOTES

Date	Description

NOTES

Date	Description

NOTES

Date	Description

NOTES

Date	Description

NOTES

Date	Description

NOTES

Date   Description

NOTES

Date	Description

NOTES

Date	Description

NOTES

Date	Description

NOTES

Date

Description

NOTES

Date	Description

NOTES

Date	Description

NOTES

Date	Description

NOTES

Date	Description

NOTES

Date	Description

NOTES

Date	Description

NOTES

Date	Description

NOTES

Date	Description

NOTES

Date	Description

NOTES

Date	Description